VIGNETTES IN PATIENT SAFETY - VOLUME 4

Edited by **Stanislaw P. Stawicki**
and **Michael S. Firstenberg**

Vignettes in Patient Safety - Volume 4
http://dx.doi.org/10.5772/intechopen.75373
Edited by Stanislaw P. Stawicki and Michael S. Firstenberg

Contributors

Margarida Eiras, Carina Silva, Ana Escoval, Vasiliki Kapaki, Daniel Ojuka, Lydia Okutoyi, Frederick Otieno, Stanislaw P. Stawicki, Parampreet Kaur, Kathryn Colonna Worrilow

First published in London, United Kingdom, 2019 by IntechOpen
IntechOpen is the global imprint of INTECHOPEN LIMITED, registered in England and Wales, registration number: 11086078, The Shard, 25th floor, 32 London Bridge Street
London, SE19SG – United Kingdom
Printed in Croatia

British Library Cataloguing-in-Publication Data
A catalogue record for this book is available from the British Library

Additional hard and PDF copies can be obtained from orders@intechopen.com

Vignettes in Patient Safety - Volume 4, Edited by Stanislaw P. Stawicki and Michael S. Firstenberg
p. cm.
Print ISBN 978-1-83962-201-4
Online ISBN 978-1-83962-202-1
eBook (PDF) ISBN 978-1-83962-203-8

For EU product safety concerns:
IN TECH d.o.o., Prolaz Marije Krucifikse Kozulić 3, 51000 Rijeka, Croatia,
info@intechopen.com or visit our website at intechopen.com.

Meet the editors

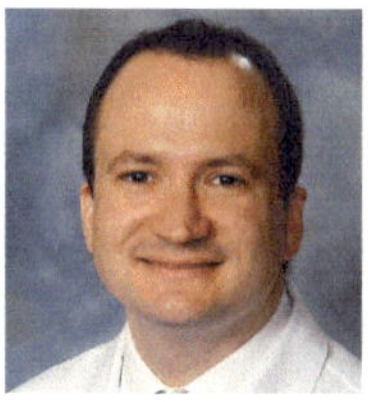

Stanislaw P. Stawicki, MD, MBA, FACS, FAIM, is Chair of the Department of Research of Innovation, St. Luke's University Health Network, Bethlehem, Pennsylvania. He is Associate Professor of Surgery at Temple University School of Medicine. Dr. Stawicki has coauthored more than 560 scholarly publications, edited more than 15 books, and is a member of multiple editorial boards. He is an expert in clinical research, health security, medical education, patient safety, traumatology, and surgical critical care. He has given numerous scientific presentations on three continents and is board certified in general surgery, surgical critical care, and neurocritical care.

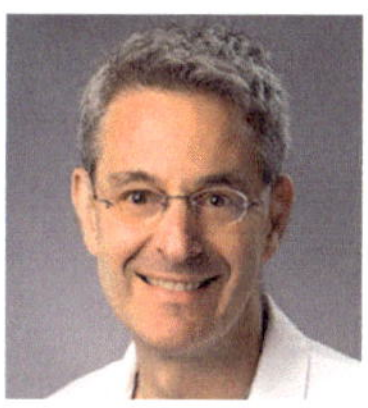

Michael S. Firstenberg, MD, FACC, FAIM, is a board-certified thoracic surgeon practicing adult cardiac surgery at the Medical Center of Aurora (Colorado, USA) where he serves as the Chief of Cardiothoracic and Vascular Surgery. He currently holds adjunct appointments in the Colleges of Medicine and Graduate Studies at Northeast Ohio Medical University and serves on the teaching faculty at the Rocky Vista University. He attended Case Western Reserve University Medical School, received his general surgery training at university hospitals in Cleveland, and completed a Fellowship in Thoracic Surgery at the Ohio State University. He also obtained advanced training in heart failure surgical therapies at the Cleveland Clinic. He is an active member of the Society of Thoracic Surgeons, American Association of Thoracic Surgeons, American College of Cardiology, and American College of Academic International Medicine (for which he is a Founding Fellow). He currently serves as Chair of the American College of Cardiology Credentialing and Member Services Committee as well as being active on several other national society committees. He is the author of well over 200 peer-reviewed manuscripts, abstracts, and book chapters. He has edited several textbooks on topics ranging from medical leadership, patient safety, endocarditis, and extracorporeal membrane oxygenation, all of which include topics that he has lectured on worldwide.

Contents

Preface

This book represents the fourth—and the last—volume of *Vignettes in Patient Safety*. Since 2017, the year of the initial publication of Volume 1, we noted significant and sustained interest in the content published in the subsequent second and third volumes. In total, the first three volumes were downloaded more than 12,000 times, with more than 50 attributable scholarly citations. This tremendous success—and validation of our efforts to promote patient safety—compelled us to embark on the current installment.

The interest in patient safety continues to grow across the world, as evidenced by the emergence of various advocacy movements and the sustained focus on improving treatment outcomes while eliminating any and all potentially preventable complications. Once again, we are very proud to play a small part in raising awareness of this critically important—and rapidly developing—area of clinical expertise. As we emphasize all of the "positives" we must remain humble and focused because much more work remains ahead of us.

When assessing the first three volumes of the *Vignettes* for any potential content gaps, we identified a number of topics that often become overlooked when it comes to general patient safety discourse. For example, the current volume contains chapters focusing on radiation monitoring and safety; primary care considerations; alarm fatigue; complications of peripheral intravenous catheters; as well as the importance of air purification systems to improving patient outcomes (and safety) through reducing the risk of healthcare associated infections. With the goal of "zero incidence" for many of the so-called "never events" there continues to be more room for improvement. As the reader will find throughout this final volume of *Vignettes in Patient Safety*, the need to develop, encourage, and support safer healthcare systems is at the core of building better hospitals and clinics of tomorrow.

Similar to the first three volumes, we utilized a case-based approach, focusing on practical aspects of identification and remediation of medical errors, including their root causes and preventive strategies. We found that by providing our readers with realistic, case-based scenarios, we empower the audience to better incorporate the educational content in their daily patient care activities. Through the use of hypothetical scenarios that are based on typical "patterns of errors," each chapter highlights its own set of unique circumstances leading to "patient harm" events. At the same time, we are able to more effectively focus the reader's attention on opportunities for improvement in bedside care delivery, clinical team interactions, regulatory considerations, and pertinent system-based processes. We hope that our audience, once equipped with this important knowledge, will be better positioned to continually reduce the ever-present risk of medical error in their clinical practices.

Another important component of the case-based approach to patient safety is the realization that as healthcare providers we do not—and should not—function in silos. Rather, we operate in an increasingly complex regulatory and clinical environment, characterized by a rapidly evolving set of expectations and competing priorities. Thus, the impact of the smallest of "adverse occurrences" within such an intricate system—despite being seemingly "insignificant" at first—

can result in both substantial and unpredictable impacts on downstream patient outcomes. Yet despite numerous challenges and opportunities, we remain optimistic that the current system-wide efforts to provide safer patient care are beginning to demonstrate tangible results.

As noted throughout this entire series, the process of assessing and evaluating patient safety events has evolved beyond "placing blame" and is now firmly focused on identifying "how and why" a specific set of events took place. Within this broader context, the overall emphasis has shifted toward proactively and constructively identifying various opportunities for improvement, instituting appropriate remedies, as well as investing in education and patient safety advocacy.

The editors of *Vignettes in Patient Safety* would like to acknowledge the tremendous efforts of all of the people involved in bringing this entire book cycle to fruition. We want to thank our friends and family who unconditionally supported this important endeavor. We must also formally acknowledge and express our appreciation to all of the authors who contributed their valuable time, experience, and effort to the *Vignettes*. Their efforts, especially in the context of an open source publication model in which the authors support the expenses of a publication, clearly reflect true dedication to the primary objectives of this book series—and willingness to share and promote this work's noble message.

The institutional development of a culture and climate focused on patient safety can be very difficult to achieve and can be frustrating to those who are truly committed to such efforts. Yet the growing number of healthcare safety champions, whose vision is to continually improve patient outcomes through individual and institutional culture change, continue unimpeded on their quest to achieving better and safer clinics, hospitals, and pharmacies around the world. One form of such championship is the willingness to share experiences and knowledge through authoring scholarly works in the form of articles and chapters. Finally, we must recognize the important role of various departments and institutions in this publication effort, both through their support of faculty time and effort, as well as through generous contributions to the open access publication process. It is only through such collaborative undertakings that we will be able to fulfill our shared goal of promoting patient safety efforts worldwide.

As we complete this final volume of *Vignettes in Patient Safety*, we hope that the collective efforts of more than 60 authors, spanning more than three years, and resulting in 40 unique vignette-based chapters, will provide our readers with important and actionable knowledge that will remain relevant for years to come. As in earlier volumes, we would like to emphasize once more that sharing one's knowledge and experiences, with the goal of helping others and making a difference, constitutes the highest form of giving. On behalf of our entire team of patient safety champions and experts, we would like to thank you!

Stanislaw P. Stawicki, MD, MBA, FACS, FAIM
Department of Research of Innovation
St. Luke's University Health Network
Bethlehem, Pennsylvania, USA

Michael S. Firstenberg, MD, FACC, FAIM
The Medical Center of Aurora
Colorado, USA

Chapter 1

Introductory Chapter: Patient Safety is the Cornerstone of Modern Health-Care Delivery Systems

Stanislaw P. Stawicki, Alyssa M. Green, Gary G. Lu,
Gregory Domer, Timothy Oskin and
Michael S. Firstenberg

Additional information is available at the end of the chapter

http://dx.doi.org/10.5772/intechopen.83842

1. Introduction

Patient safety (PS) is inextricably linked to quality of care. In the value-driven paradigm of modern health-care systems, focus on these critical elements is required for institutions wishing to stay relevant and competitive [1–5]. This is the fourth and final volume of the **Vignettes in Patient Safety**. The previous three volumes featured a total of 31 chapters, covering a multitude of topics in PS and related fields. Discussed among a variety of concepts were PS education, institutional culture, application of evidence-based practices, handoff communication, disruptive behaviors, fatigue and burnout, team collaboration, and a plethora of discipline-specific topics [5–7]. The current book adds eight additional chapters, including in-depth discussions on communication, medication errors, patient safety culture, alarm fatigue, radiation safety, complications of intravenous therapy, as well as health-care policy and operations.

What has become clear over the course of the four volumes of the **Vignettes in Patient Safety** is that, despite continuous long-term efforts by health-care systems to enhance PS, numerous opportunities for improvement remain. In fact, we are all too often faced with the reality that our still limited knowledge of various gaps in safety, including any associated errors and consequences, can affect patient quality of life, the overall trust in our health-care systems, as well as health-care expenses overall [5, 8, 9]. Slowly and methodically, our understanding of how individuals, teams, and systems can more effectively prevent errors continues to evolve. With the advent of electronic medical records, the ability to capture critical events and their timing made it possible to construct root cause analyses more effectively and accurately, further accelerating our understanding of various "gaps in safety" and corresponding "failure modes" [10–12]. It is hoped that these incremental steps will collectively help reduce both the frequency and impact of medical errors and hopefully lead to better mitigation strategies and the ultimate attainment of the elusive "zero incidence" goal [13]. Some examples of early successes include the growing evidence that adverse outcomes are becoming less common across different areas of care, likely due to a combination of better training and more effective processes and procedures becoming integrated into existing safety systems [11, 14–16]. Concepts such as "failure to rescue" and "never-events" serve to focus teams on minimizing relatively infrequent, but often catastrophic events (e.g., hospital acquired infections; delays in therapy for critical diagnoses such as stroke, sepsis, acute respiratory failure, or acute myocardial infarction) [17–20]. Again, the ultimate goal is to simultaneously achieve 100% readiness and 0% incidence for any such occurrences.

The evolving role of public reporting of quality and safety data, including various clinical metrics and outcomes, will provide a powerful stimulus for developing processes and systems that will make patient care both safer and more efficient [21, 22]. However, without proper organizational and individual context, exclusive attention to such metrics will not inherently result in better or safer care [23–25]. For example, a study looking at 28 strategies to improve "door-to-balloon time" (a commonly utilized quality metric in cardiovascular medicine) across 365 hospitals demonstrated that despite several strategies being associated with substantial reductions in "door-to-balloon time," only a minority of institutions was actually utilizing these proven approaches [26]. It is therefore critically important to evaluate PS systems in a comprehensive and multifactorial fashion, maintaining open and constructive stance on exploring "what is going right", "what has gone wrong", and "what might go wrong."

2. Integrative approach to patient safety

The success of patient safety initiatives and corresponding systemic implementations is heavily dependent on the thorough understanding of the overall framework within which structures, processes, and outcomes dynamically interact in health-care [27]. With that knowledge, it is important to integrate key processes in order to increase organizational efficiency and effectiveness. Examples of successful interventions that span across different domains of the health-care matrix include checklists, standardized handoff protocols, intense analyses/sentinel event reviews, and institutional safety and quality improvement projects [5, 7, 28].

Using specialized processes, such as the plan-do-check-act (PDCA) quality improvement cycle, modern PS protocols and approaches continue to evolve and become increasingly more optimized [29]. Organizations must continue to transform PS systems into more horizontal, cross-disciplinary platforms that function in a nonpunitive, fair, respectful, and inclusive fashion [30, 31]. Determinations regarding the importance and relevance of any constructive input should not be based on hierarchical considerations, but rather on the informational content being communicated [28, 32, 33]. The end goal is to hard-wire quality and safety improvement into the fabric of health-care operations, both clinical and nonclinical [33]. To paraphrase, there should be a constant emphasis on ensuring that dedicated institutional processes are focused on making it easy to "do the right thing" and harder to "do the wrong thing." The use of checklists helps facilitate just that. Standardization of the process by incorporating all critical steps into an easy-to-follow framework provides a potent fail-safe measure to prevent both human and systemic errors [34, 35].

Of importance, continuous real-time review of patient safety and quality processes must be performed to ensure that all active implementations are being monitored for proper functioning, as well as any unintended consequences or down-stream problems, for either the patient or the health-care system [29, 36, 37]. This can be accomplished through conducting regular performance improvement initiatives, hiring dedicated staff to track and report on different quality measures, and building robust systems to ensure not only that safety and quality are being upheld but also to resolve any issues as they arise [7, 38]. For example, there are numerous initiatives to reduce the incidence of deep vein thrombosis and pulmonary embolisms [39–41]. Clearly, such initiatives are intended to address a substantial and highly complex set of PS issues. Yet, it is critical for clinicians to avoid "blindly" following protocols and guidelines that rely solely on "guaranteeing" that every patient is receiving "standard of care" anticoagulation prophylaxis while failing to consider the potential impact of anticoagulation on bleeding and related complications. Similarly, patients who are fully ambulatory are much less likely to benefit from antithrombotic prophylaxis than patients who are tethered to their beds and unlikely to ambulate for three or more days. Finally, clinicians must always be sensitive to the impact of therapeutic anticoagulation under circumstances where risks outweigh benefits of such intervention [42]. Use of clinical judgment is imperative in such situations in order to determine the necessity, applicability, and appropriateness of any evidence-based protocol or guideline.

3. Gradual and sustainable culture change

Patient safety culture depends heavily on institutional ability to create an environment that welcomes honest disclosure and constructive, nonjudgmental feedback [43]. It has been shown that more positive PS culture correlates with fewer adverse health-care events [44]. A change in culture is no easy feat, but it is instrumental in the development of an environment that does not penalize human error (**Figure 1**). It has been suggested that although humans certainly contribute to adverse events, faulty organizational systems are more likely to be at the root of many of these errors [45]. This suggests that a more fundamental change is needed to affect the safety and quality of care delivered within the health-care system. It has been pointed out that institutions fully committed to a culture of patient safety have seen reductions in medical errors [45]. This involves integration of "error management strategies" to analyze the causes of error and instituting mechanisms of prevention [46]. Buy-in from administration as well as other leadership is integral to the process of adoption of a patient safety culture. Without engagement from leadership, it will be difficult to transform existing organizational "patterns and habits". Hospital leadership must set PS as a priority, even

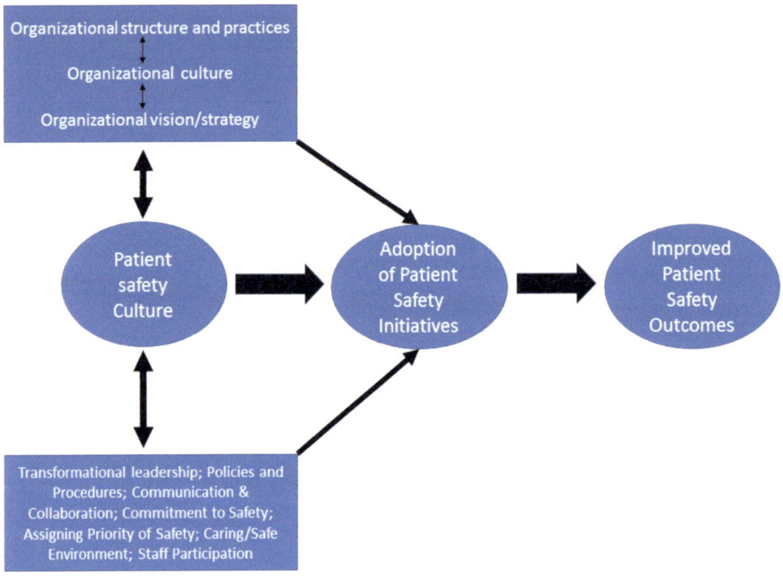

Figure 1. The relationship between institutional culture of safety and improved patient outcomes involves the presence of key foundational factors coupled with effective adoption of patient safety initiatives and the fostering of constructive feedback.

placing it above clinical productivity [45]. Institutional leaders are instrumental in creating a culture of honest disclosure, support, and constructive feedback. When errors occur, root cause analysis ensues to understand which specific systemic factors may have been contributory. The natural inclination to point fingers and blame a specific person or persons for making a mistake is discouraged. Adjustments to the system are then implemented to prevent the reoccurrence of the specific error in question. This includes sitting down with the individuals involved and addressing what went wrong and what needs to be done to prevent similar errors in the future. An action plan may include instituting failsafe mechanisms within the system to prevent performance of certain harmful actions. Development of a patient safety culture depends heavily on organizational structure and priorities, transformational leadership that can trickle down to other stakeholders as well as effective communication amongst all parties involved. Taken collectively, all of the above interventions act synergistically to help create and reinforce a culture of patient safety.

Once safe systems are in place, their preservation becomes critical. In addition, the long-term goal then transitions into permanent culture change that hopefully becomes a source of pride for both employees and the organization [7, 28]. Once a culture of safety is achieved, other aspects of institutional change can occur, including alignment of goals, especially between clinicians and administration. By association, one can also expect improved employee morale, enhanced quality of care, and other positive manifestations of a well-functioning organization. As a word of caution, the same can also occur "in reverse," where negative influences can insidiously and gradually erode various positive elements and influences within the institutional culture [7, 47–50].

4. The challenge of habits: The art of learning and unlearning

A culture of safety represents a complex system of behaviors and hardwired procedures, designed to synergistically create a safe, reliable and efficient, high-quality clinical environment [51, 52]. The creation of such a sophisticated institutional cultural milieu requires all stakeholders to commit to unprecedented amounts of commitment and flexibility [51–53]. In many cases, the organizational transition process can span years and require the replacement of "bad habits" with positive behaviors—a difficult undertaking given the inherent human tendency to resist change when having to "unlearn things" [54]. So how do we change bad habits, motivate people to "do the right thing", and sustainably instill safe and productive behaviors? To motivate individuals, we must first recognize why and how people are influenced. In his book *Drive: The Surprising Truth About What Motivates Us*, Daniel Pink points out that historically our good behavior has been incentivized with rewards and our bad behaviors reprimanded [55]. This carries the unintended consequence of undermining an individual's motivation. He suggests humans have a strong inner-drive to be autonomous, self-determined, and connected. We all seek the trifecta of attaining autonomy, mastery, and purpose in both our work and our lives. Upon achieving these elements, people will take on greater responsibility, believing they are effecting positive change. With this sense of autonomy and purpose comes increased self-esteem, confidence, and motivation to go beyond what is merely required. The pursuit of mastery naturally follows [55].

5. The importance of anonymous event reporting in maintaining patient safety

In many countries, incident reporting in health-care has become a well-accepted method of improving overall patient safety [56]. Strategic collection of adverse events and "near misses" from across our care delivery platforms allows safety specialists to efficiently analyze each event, identify potential underlying factors, and implement action plans based on this knowledge to help reduce systemic risk levels in the future [5, 7]. However, in the United States, medical errors continue to be significantly underreported, as exemplified in a study of over 1600 hospitals which concluded that substantial proportion of facilities lacked adequate event reporting systems [57].

The overarching question then becomes, which components comprise a thorough, accurate, and effective reporting system design within health-care? Specifically, published studies identify several factors that are essential to constructive "incident reporting". These factors include: staff willingness to report incidents, removal of barriers to incident reporting, the overall culture surrounding reporting, classifying and monitoring the number of incidents reported, taxonomies for various types of patient safety events, and the constitution of incident reporting systems [58–60]. Moreover, one of the greatest challenges that exist with regards to the incident reporting process is determining a way to create a "no blame" culture and balancing team accountability versus individual responsibility [58–60].

Presently, reporting systems within health-care tend to place greater emphasis on collecting reports than on conducting advanced analyses and identifying learning opportunities that can be gleaned from the available wealth of information [61–63]. One study suggests that systems should focus on providing health-care professionals with feedback pertaining to incidents that occurred, including any action(s) taken, to then serve as an integral part of the cycle of continuous improvement and the creation of a culture of safety [64]. Health-care workers who feel protected by employers after disclosing an incident, primarily through anonymity, generally are more likely to report the event through established mechanisms, and the reported event can then be utilized as a constructive example for all staff in regards to reducing risks and embracing PS measures. In summary, appropriately structured, anonymous event reporting programs have contributed to significant changes in practices, including new care processes, constructive behavioral changes, as well as more realistic risk perception and awareness of the importance of a culture of safety.

6. Topics in the current book

The current text contains some unique and perhaps under-appreciated topics. Beginning with "anatomy of medication errors", there are unique chapters on patient safety culture in primary care practices, PS perspectives in the context of health-care operations and risk management, alarm fatigue, the importance of air filtration systems, and even medical radiation safety (both diagnostic and therapeutic). Although seemingly diverse and unrelated, the common thread among the chapters of this final volume of **The Vignettes** is the continued demonstration of the critical importance of teamwork within our increasingly complex health-care systems. Again highlighted are the key elements of communication, collaboration, and coordination [65–67].

7. Conclusion

As our Editorial Team's journey through the four volumes of **The Vignettes in Patient Safety** comes to an end, we hope that our primary goals of increasing awareness and providing clinically applicable solutions toward enhancing PS have been accomplished satisfactorily. In addition, what both the editors and authors have recognized is how many more opportunities there are to better understand the challenges of creating and preserving an institutional culture that is truly focused on patient safety. Without a doubt, and unfortunately, there could be many more volumes on this topic to help illustrate how complex the current PS environment has become—and how many opportunities for improvement still exist. It is easy to become discouraged when one reads and analyzes PS vignettes throughout the four volumes, realizing that it is sometimes only by accident and luck that satisfactory clinical results are achieved. At the same time, one must appreciate and be amazed at - especially given the complexity of modern health-care environment - how much more frequently things go right and patients get better.

Author details

Stanislaw P. Stawicki[1]*, Alyssa M. Green[1], Gary G. Lu[2], Gregory Domer[3], Timothy Oskin[3] and Michael S. Firstenberg[4]

*Address all correspondence to: stawicki.ace@gmail.com

1 Department of Research and Innovation, St. Luke's University Health Network, Bethlehem, Pennsylvania, USA

2 Department of Medicine, Section of Hematology and Oncology, St. Luke's University Health Network, Bethlehem, Pennsylvania, USA

3 Department of Surgery, Division of Vascular Surgery, St. Luke's University Health Network, Bethlehem, Pennsylvania, USA

4 Department of Surgery (Cardiothoracic), The Medical Center of Aurora, Aurora, Colorado, USA

References

[1] Nerenz D, Neil N. Performance Measures for Health Care Systems. Commissioned Paper for the Center for Health Management Research. 2001

[2] Berwick DM, Nolan TW, Whittington J. The triple aim: Care, health, and cost. Health Affairs. 2008;**27**(3):759-769

[3] Groenewoud A. Value Based Competition in Health Care. A Critical Reflection from an Ethical Point of View. 2015

[4] Roush T. Pay for Performance on Quality of Health Care Justified Transition? 2013

[5] Stawicki SP, Firstenberg MS. Introductory chapter: The decades long quest continues toward better, safer healthcare systems. In: Vignettes in Patient Safety-Volume 1. Rijeka: InTech; 2017

[6] Stawicki SP, Firstenberg MS. Vignettes in Patient Safety. Vol. 3. London, England: IntechOpen; 2018

[7] Tolentino JC et al. Introductory chapter: Developing patient safety champions. In: Vignettes in Patient Safety. Vol. 2. Rijeka: InTech; 2018

[8] Wachter RM. Patient safety at ten: Unmistakable progress, troubling gaps. Health Affairs. 2009;**29**(1):165-173

[9] Becher EC, Chassin MR. Improving quality, minimizing error: Making it happen. Health Affairs. 2001;**20**(3):68-81

[10] Shortell SM, Bennett CL, Byck GR. Assessing the impact of continuous quality improvement on clinical practice: What it will take to accelerate progress. The Milbank Quarterly. 1998;**76**(4):593-624

[11] Hatry HP. Performance Measurement: Getting Results. Washington, DC: The Urban Institute Press; 2006

[12] Kaldjian LC et al. Reporting medical errors to improve patient safety: A survey of physicians in teaching hospitals. Archives of Internal Medicine. 2008;**168**(1):40-46

[13] Nguyen MC, Moffatt-Bruce SD. What's new in academic medicine? Retained surgical items: Is "zero incidence" achievable? International Journal of Academic Medicine. 2016;**2**(1):1

[14] Clark SL et al. Improved outcomes, fewer cesarean deliveries, and reduced litigation: Results of a new paradigm in patient safety. American Journal of Obstetrics and Gynecology. 2008;**199**(2):105.e1-105.e7

[15] de Vries EN et al. Effect of a comprehensive surgical safety system on patient outcomes. New England Journal of Medicine. 2010;**363**(20):1928-1937

[16] Pronovost PJ et al. Improving patient safety in intensive care units in Michigan. Journal of Critical Care. 2008;**23**(2):207-221

[17] Pucher P. Structural and Care Process Improvement of Ward-based Postoperative Care to Optimise Surgical Outcomes. 2014

[18] Nye AI. Experience of Nurses in Caring for Patients with Short Term Indwelling Urinary Catheters during Hospitalization: A Challenge to Reshape Caring Practices. Pullman, WA: Washington State University; 2018

[19] Tichansky DS, Morton J, Jones DB. The SAGES manual of quality, outcomes and patient safety. New York, NY: Springer Science & Business Media; 2011

[20] Burnett S, Norris B, Flin R. Never events: The cultural and systems issues that cannot be addressed by individual action plans. Clinical Risk. 2012;**18**(6):213-216

[21] Goode LD et al. When is "good enough"? The role and responsibility of physicians to improve patient safety. Academic Medicine. 2002;**77**(10):947-952

[22] Furrow BR. Regulating patient safety: The patient protection and affordable care act. University of Pennsylvania Law Review. 2010;**159**:1727

[23] Shojania KG et al. Making health care safer: A critical analysis of patient safety practices. Evidence Report/Technology Assessment (Summary). 2001;**43**(1):668

[24] Leape LL, Berwick DM, Bates DW. What practices will most improve safety?: Evidence-based medicine meets patient safety. JAMA. 2002;**288**(4):501-507

[25] Shojania KG et al. Safe but sound: Patient safety meets evidence-based medicine. JAMA. 2002;**288**(4):508-513

[26] Bradley EH et al. Strategies for reducing the door-to-balloon time in acute myocardial infarction. New England Journal of Medicine. 2006;**355**(22):2308-2320

[27] Carayon P et al. Work system design for patient safety: The SEIPS model. BMJ Quality and Safety. 2006;**15**(suppl 1):i50-i58

[28] Stawicki S et al. Fundamentals of Patient Safety in Medicine and Surgery. New Delhi: Wolters Kluwer Health (India) Pvt Ltd; 2014

[29] Saeed M et al. Fact versus conjecture: Exploring levels of evidence in the context of patient safety and care quality. In: Vignettes in Patient Safety. Vol. 3. Rijeka: IntechOpen; 2018

[30] Hannawa AF et al. Building bridges: Future directions for medical error disclosure research. Patient Education and Counseling. 2013;**92**(3):319-327

[31] Patankar MS. Safety culture: Building and sustaining a cultural change in aviation and healthcare. Burlington, VT: Ashgate Publishing, Ltd; 2012

[32] Lewis GH et al. Counterheroism, common knowledge, and ergonomics: Concepts from aviation that could improve patient safety. The Milbank Quarterly. 2011;**89**(1):4-38

[33] Sehgal NL et al. A multidisciplinary teamwork training program: The Triad for Optimal Patient Safety (TOPS) experience. Journal of General Internal Medicine. 2008;**23**(12): 2053-2057

[34] Macdonald D. Practical Industrial Safety, Risk Assessment and Shutdown Systems. Burlington, MA: Elsevier; 2003

[35] Smith E et al. Surgical safety checklist: Productive, nondisruptive, and the "right thing to do". Journal of Postgraduate Medicine. 2015;**61**(3):214

[36] Croskerry P, Cosby KS. Patient Safety in Emergency Medicine. Philadelphia, PA: Lippincott Williams & Wilkins; 2009

[37] Martinez EA, Buck AMVDW. Quality Improvement and Patient Safety. In: Miller RD, Cohen NH, Eriksson LI, et al. Philadelphia, PA: Elsevier; pp. 87-105

[38] Ponte PR, Peterson K. A patient-and family-centered care model paves the way for a culture of quality and safety. Critical Care Nursing Clinics of North America. 2008;**20**(4): 451-464

[39] Beckman MG et al. Venous thromboembolism: A public health concern. American Journal of Preventive Medicine. 2010;**38**(4):S495-S501

[40] Michota FA. Bridging the gap between evidence and practice in venous thromboembolism prophylaxis: The quality improvement process. Journal of General Internal Medicine. 2007;**22**(12):1762-1770

[41] Stawicki SP et al. Deep venous thrombosis and pulmonary embolism in trauma patients: An overstatement of the problem? The American Surgeon. 2005;**71**(5):387-391

[42] Hon H et al. Inappropriate preinjury warfarin use in trauma patients: A call for a safety initiative. Journal of Postgraduate Medicine. 2016;**62**(2):73

[43] Nieva V, Sorra J. Safety culture assessment: A tool for improving patient safety in healthcare organizations. BMJ Quality and Safety. 2003;**12**(suppl 2):ii17-ii23

[44] Mardon RE et al. Exploring relationships between hospital patient safety culture and adverse events. Journal of Patient Safety. 2010;**6**(4):226-232

[45] McFadden KL, Henagan SC, Gowen CR III. The patient safety chain: Transformational leadership's effect on patient safety culture, initiatives, and outcomes. Journal of Operations Management. 2009;**27**(5):390-404

[46] Helmreich RL. On error management: Lessons from aviation. BMJ. 2000;**320**(7237):781-785

[47] Prilleltensky I, Prilleltensky O. Promoting Well-being: Linking Personal, Organizational, and Community Change. Hoboken, NJ: John Wiley & Sons; 2007

[48] Katcher BL, Snyder A. 30 Reasons Employees Hate Their Managers: What Your People May be Thinking and What You Can Do about it. New York, NY: AMACOM/American Management Association; 2007

[49] Roffey S. Introduction to positive relationships: Evidence-based practice across the world. In: Positive Relationships. Springer; 2012. pp. 1-15

[50] Tolentino JC et al. What's new in academic medicine: Can we effectively address the burnout epidemic in healthcare? International Journal of Academic Medicine. 2017;**3**(3):1

[51] Cochrane BS et al. High reliability in healthcare: Creating the culture and mindset for patient safety. In: Healthcare Management Forum. Los Angeles, CA: SAGE Publications Sage CA; 2017

[52] Cochrane BS et al. Back to the future: Patient experience and the link to quality, safety, and financial performance. In: Healthcare Management Forum. Los Angeles, CA: SAGE Publications Sage CA; 2015

[53] Stawicki SPA, Firstenberg MS. Fundamentals of Leadership for Healthcare Professionals. Hauppauge, NY: NOVA Science Publishers; 2018. p. 287

[54] Carroll AE. It's Hard for Doctors to Unlearn Things. That's Costly for All of Us. 2018. Available from: https://www.nytimes.com/2018/09/10/upshot/its-hard-for-doctors-to-unlearn-things-thats-costly-for-all-of-us.html [Accessed: 13-10-2018]

[55] Pink DH. Drive: The Surprising Truth about What Motivates Us. New York, NY: Penguin; 2011

[56] Vincent C. Reporting and Learning Systems. Patient Safety. 2nd ed. Chichester: Wiley Blackwell; 2010. pp. 75-95

[57] Evans SM et al. Attitudes and barriers to incident reporting: A collaborative hospital study. BMJ Quality and Safety. 2006;**15**(1):39-43

[58] Wilson KA et al. Promoting health care safety through training high reliability teams. BMJ Quality and Safety. 2005;**14**(4):303-309

[59] Espin S et al. Persistence of unsafe practice in everyday work: An exploration of organizational and psychological factors constraining safety in the operating room. BMJ Quality and Safety. 2006;**15**(3):165-170

[60] Donaldson MS, Corrigan JM, Kohn LT. To Err is Human: Building a Safer Health System. Vol. 6. Washington, DC: National Academies Press; 2000

[61] Battles JB et al. The attributes of medical event-reporting systems. Archives of Pathology & Laboratory Medicine. 1998;**122**(3):132-138

[62] Wu AW, Pronovost P, Morlock L. ICU incident reporting systems. Journal of Critical Care. 2002;**17**(2):86-94

[63] Suresh G et al. Voluntary anonymous reporting of medical errors for neonatal intensive care. Pediatrics. 2004;**113**(6):1609-1618

[64] Clarke I. Learning from critical incidents. Advances in Psychiatric Treatment. 2008;**14**(6):460-468

[65] Mills P, Neily J, Dunn E. Teamwork and communication in surgical teams: Implications for patient safety. Journal of the American College of Surgeons. 2008;**206**(1):107-112

[66] O'Daniel M, Rosenstein AH. Professional Communication and Team Collaboration. In: Hughes RG, editor. Patient Safety and Quality: An Evidence-Based Handbook for Nurses. Rockville (MD): Agency for Healthcare Research and Quality (US); 2008 Apr. Chapter 33

[67] Dingley C, Daugherty K, Derieg MK, et al. Improving Patient Safety Through Provider Communication Strategy Enhancements. In: Henriksen K, Battles JB, Keyes MA, et al., editors. Advances in Patient Safety: New Directions and Alternative Approaches (Vol. 3: Performance and Tools). Rockville (MD): Agency for Healthcare Research and Quality (US); 2008 Aug

Chapter 2

Patient Safety Culture in Portuguese Primary Care: Validation of the Portuguese Version of the Medical Office Survey

Margarida Eiras, Ana Escoval and Carina Silva

Additional information is available at the end of the chapter

http://dx.doi.org/10.5772/intechopen.80035

Abstract

Background: Assessing patient safety culture is a strategic priority worldwide, and Portugal is no exception.

Objective: It is the objective of this work to translate, adapt, validate, and analyze the reliability of the Medical Office Survey on Patient Safety Culture in Portuguese Primary Health Care (MOSPSC).

Methods: The methodology adopted focused on transcultural translation and adaptation using the Translation Guidelines for the Agency for Healthcare Research and Quality (AHRQ) surveys on Patient Safety Culture, and reliability was conducted using Cronbach's α and average inter-item correlation. Exploratory factor analysis and confirmatory factor analysis were performed to investigate the observed data that fit to the dimensional structure proposed in the AHRQ Portuguese version.

Results: The initial sample ($n = 7299$) was submitted to a missing value analysis, obtaining a final sample of 4304 surveys. With exploratory factor analysis, it was obtained a structure with eight composites, one item was removed, and several items moved to other composites. With confirmatory factor analysis, one composite was removed. For both proposed model structures, good results were achieved for goodness of fit indices.

Conclusions: The Portuguese version of the MOSPSC resulted in nine composites with good reliability and construct validity.

Keywords: patient safety, primary care, safety culture, validity, reliability, exploratory factor analysis, confirmatory factor analysis

1. Introduction

Health care is vulnerable to error, and so all health care environments and professionals are involved in complex care processes. Since the IOM report [1], almost all countries and health care organizations are attending to Patient Safety issues. In more recent years, the European Council launched a recommendation [2] that shows the importance of establishing patient safety culture in all health care settings. We can read in this recommendation that a poor patient safety represents both a severe public health problem and a high economic burden on limited health resources. A large proportion of adverse events, both in the hospital sector and in primary care, are preventable with systemic factors appearing to account for a majority of them.

Before implementing patient safety programs, health care staff must understand their safety culture [3]. Quantitative instruments designed to assess safety culture have been developed, and a few review articles have been published, which allows a more comprehensive way of implementing models of safety culture [4]. Measuring health care safety culture enables us to identify improvements, safety behaviors, and outcomes for both patients and staff. These instruments should also serve as decision making tools, especially for managers.

Much has been done in hospital environment, and more recently, primary care has also been in the sights. A few review articles were published allowing researchers and primary care staff to take robust decisions on tools to assess patient safety culture [5–7].

With the publication of the National Patient Safety Plan (2015–2020), the Portuguese Directory of Health along with the Portuguese Hospital Association carried out patient safety culture assessment either in hospitals or in primary care. It was published as a national standard, and every 2 years, patient safety culture is assessed either in primary care or in hospitals nationwide.

The purpose of this study was to translate, adapt, validate, and analyze the reliability and validity of the Portuguese version of the Medical Office Survey on Patient Safety Culture.

2. Methods

2.1. Medical Office Survey on Patient Safety Culture

The Medical Office Survey on Patient Safety Culture (MOSPSC) is a self-administered tool, which was developed by the Agency for Healthcare Research and Quality (AHRQ) in 2007 [8], and is designed specifically for outpatient medical office providers and other staff and asks for their opinions about the culture of patient safety and health care quality in their medical offices. Although in Portugal the health system is completely different than in the United States, we considered that the primary care environment and culture are similar, which lead us to test its use.

This survey has 38 items grouped into 10 composites and includes questions that ask respondents about problems related to exchange information with other settings and about access to care. Respondents are also asked to rate their medical office in five areas of health care quality (patient centered, effective, timely, efficient, and equitable) and to provide an overall rating on patient safety (**Table 1**).

Composites	Items
1. Teamwork	C1; C2; C5; C13
2. Patient Care Tracking/Follow Up	D3; D5; D6; D9
3. Organizational Learning	F1; F5; F7
4. Overall Perceptions of Patient Safety and Quality	F2; F3; F4R; F6R
5. Staff Training	C4; C7; C10R
6. Owner/Managing Partner/Leadership Support for Patient Safety	E1R; E2R; E3; E4R
7. Communication about Error	D7R; D8R; D11; D12
8. Communication Openness	D1; D2; D4R; D10R
9. Office Processes and Standardization	C8R; C9; C12R; C15
10. Work Pressure and Pace	C3R; C6R; C11; C14R

Table 1. MOSPSC composites and items.

According to the MOSPSC author's [8], patient safety culture composites and its definitions are:

1. Teamwork—the extent to which the office has a culture of teamwork, mutual respect, and close working relationships among staff and providers.

2. Patient Care Tracking/Follow Up—the extent to which the office reminds patients about appointments, documents how well patients follow treatment plans, follows up with patients who need monitoring, and follows up when reports from an outside provider are not received.

3. Organizational Learning—the extent to which the office has a learning culture that facilitates making changes in office processes to improve the quality of patient care and evaluates changes for effectiveness.

4. Overall Perceptions of Patient Safety and Quality—the extent to which the quality of patient care is more important than getting more work done, office processes are good at preventing mistakes, and mistakes do not happen more than they should.

5. Staff Training—the extent to the office gives providers and staff effective on-the-job training, trains them on new processes, and does not assign tasks they have not been trained to perform.

6. Owner/Managing Partner/Leadership Support for Patient Safety—the extent to which office leadership actively supports quality and patient safety, places a high priority on improving patient care processes, does not overlook mistakes, and makes decisions based on what is best for patients.

7. Communication about Error—the extent to which providers and staff are willing to report mistakes they observe and do not feel like their mistakes are held against them, and

providers and staff talk openly about office problems and how to prevent errors from happening.

8. Communication Openness—the extent to which providers in the office are open to staff ideas about how to improve office processes, and staff are encouraged to express alternative viewpoints and do not find it difficult to voice disagreement.
9. Office Processes and Standardization—the extent to which the office is organized, has an effective workflow, has standardized processes for completing tasks, and has good procedures for checking the accuracy of work performed.
10. Work Pressure and Pace—the extent to which there are enough staff and providers to handle the patient load, and the office work pace is not hectic.

Since the publication of the National Patient Safety Plan (2015–2020), the Portuguese Directory of Health along with the Portuguese Hospital Association carried out patient safety culture assessment either in hospitals or in primary care. For this purpose, the MOSPSC was the chosen tool because [8]:

- it raises provider and staff awareness about patient safety;
- it assesses the current status of patient safety culture;
- it identifies strengths and areas for patient safety culture improvement;
- it examines trends in patient safety culture change over time;
- it evaluates the cultural impact of patient safety initiatives and interventions;
- it conducts comparisons within and across organizations;
- it has been used in several countries in Europe (which makes benchmark possible) [9, 10], and the results of the LINEUS study [9] show that it is useful and applicable to assess patient safety culture at primary health care services in Europe.

The European Society for Quality and Safety in Family Practice (EQuiP) and the World Family Doctors. Caring for People (WONCA Europe) [11] conducted a study to spread the MOSPSC among EQuiP delegates, explore their views and opinions on the MOSPSC, and explore with them the feasibility of the MOSPSC among European countries. Nineteen countries were involved, and 63% of respondents find it would be interesting to use MOSPSC.

2.2. Translation and cultural adaptation process

Immediately after author's permission for MOSPSC use, the survey was translated from English to Portuguese (T1) and backward (T2) by two independent translators, native speakers of Portuguese, and bilingual in English/Portuguese, experienced in this method and knowledgeable about the research objective (Step 1). The two versions (T1 and T2) were compared with the original version of the MOSPSC (Step 2). Back translation by two independent translators (R-T1 and R-T2) was carried out by bilingual native English, who were unfamiliar with the original version of tool and not knowledgeable about the study objectives (Step 3). Discrepancies were assessed, and the cross-cultural adaptations were undertaken (Step 4).

Content validity and semantic analysis were undertaken by six experts chosen from the primary care sector and knowledge on this topic and with research experience (Step 5).

The pretest was applied (Step 6), which was aimed at assessing whether the MOSPSC was understandable to a larger number of people in the target population. The last version of the MOSPSC was then administered in Web-based format, and we used all recommendations from AHRQ [11] to publicize and promote the survey.

The Portuguese Directory of Health published a national standard that requires patient safety culture assessment in primary care units (PCUs) nationwide (52 PCUs) every 2 years. A personalized link was sent to all PCUs, where a focal point was in charge of facilitating the administration of the survey. In order to track and maximize response rates, a link was sent to each office PCU. We sent another link so that the focal point could check response rates along the administration period, which occurred from March 16 till April 30, 2017.

2.3. Statistical analysis

Our goal was to assess the validity and reliability of the Portuguese version of the MOSPSC, by verifying if the 10 patient-safety culture composites were appropriate for the Portuguese population. The R software was used for statistical analysis, and the negatively worded items were reverse-scored and they are denoted by R letter.

Descriptive statistics were used to examine response variability and missing data. To identify and eliminate those items with missing data, an individual descriptive item analysis was performed. A missing-value analysis was performed to verify if it was necessary to remove surveys from the data set. Every survey with missing values was removed, and surveys with more than 1 response in the option "not applicable" were removed. For the remaining surveys with only one answer in option "not applicable," it was replaced by the middle category in a five-point Likert scale. An empirical rule of 10 respondents per patient safety culture item in a survey with 38 items means that at least 380 completed surveys were needed.

A reliability analysis (internal consistency) was performed using Cronbach's α, where it indicates the extent to which surveys items can be treated as a single latent construct. Values >0.7 reliability is considered adequate for a survey instrument [12], although some authors consider >0.6 adequate [13]. For the entire survey, Cronbach's α should be at least 0.9 [12]. However, the validity of this measure has been questioned, and several authors have suggested alternative measures. In this study, we also used the average inter-item correlation (AIIC), which is independent of the number of items and sample size. This measure evaluates how items within a composite correlate, i.e., there is evidence that the items are measuring the same underlying composite. A rule-of-thumb is that AIIC should be between 0.15 and 0.5 [14].

An exploratory factor analysis (EFA) was performed. EFA is a cluster of common methods used to explore the underlying pattern of relationships among multiple observed variables. EFA is useful for assessing the dimensionality of questionnaire scales that measure underlying latent variables. Researchers use EFA to hypothesize and, later, confirm, through replication or confirmatory factor analysis (CFA), the model that gave rise to the interrelationships among the scale's variables. EFA for ordinal data, a benefit over conventional criteria, where the Pearson correlation matrix is used. Pearson correlations assume that data have been measured on, at least, an equal interval scale, and a linear relationship exists between the variables. These assumptions are typically violated in the case of variables measured using ordinal rating scales. Pearson correlations have been found to underestimate the strength of relationships between ordinal items.

EFA is useful for assessing the dimensionality of survey scales that measure underlying latent variables. This factor analysis gives an indication of the number of factors that the survey appears to measure of its intended subject. In this way, through EFA, we can investigate if the Portuguese data will produce different factors from the American structure.

Since the data are ordinal, it was used a polychoric correlation matrix for EFA analysis and a Varimax rotation. To decide on the number of factors, it was used a parallel analysis [15, 16]. Items with a factor loading lower than 0.4 on all factors were excluded. Libraries *psych* and *polycor* from R were used [17, 18].

We used confirmatory factor analysis (CFA) for ordinal data to compare the Portuguese sample factor structure to the factor structure reported for the original HSOPSC. CFA for ordinal data will use diagonally weighted least squares (DWLS) to estimate the model parameters, but it will use the full weight matrix to compute robust standard errors and a mean- and variance-adjusted test statistic. We used the goodness-of-fit index (GFI), which accounts for the proportion of observed covariance between the manifest variables (items), explained by the fitted model (a concept similar to the coefficient of determination in linear regression). Generally, GFI values between 0.9 and 0.95 indicate good fit, and GFI values above 0.95 indicate a very good fit. Bentler's comparative fit index (CFI) was used to correct the underestimation that can occur when samples are small. CFI is independent from the sample size. Values between 0.9 and 0.95 indicate good fit, and values equal to or above 0.95 indicate a very good fit. The Tucker-Lewis index (TLI) varies between 0 and 1; values close to 1 indicate a good fit. Parsimony GPI (PGFI) is obtained to compensate for the "artificial" improvement in the model, which is achieved simply by adding more parameters, i.e., a more complex model may have better fit than a simpler model (parsimonious). Values between 0.6 and 0.8 indicate a reasonable fit and values above 0.8 a good fit. The index root mean square error of approximation (RMSEA) was used to adjust the model simply by adding more parameters. Empirical studies suggest that the model fit is considered good for values ranging between 0.05 and 0.08 and very good for values less than 0.05. The *lavaan* library from R was used [19].

3. Results

3.1. Demographic data

A total of 7299 respondents provided feedback (response rate of 32.2%), 38% were nurses, 27% physicians, and 19% secretary/clerk (**Table 2**).

Average composite positive responses were obtained (**Table 3**). The lowest positive scores were found in composites *Work Pressure and Pace, Owner/Managing Partner/Leadership Support for Patient Safety,* and *Staff Training.* The composites with highest scores were *Teamwork, Patient Care Tracking/Follow Up,* and *Organization Learning.*

	Respondents	
	N	%
Physicians	1954	27
Nurses	2729	38
Assistant	456	6
Secretary	1380	19
Technicians	560	7
Others	136	2
Total	7215	
Missing values	84	
Total	7299	

Table 2. Demographic characteristics.

Composite	Average positive responses (%)
1. Teamwork	76
2. Patient Care Tracking/Follow Up	76
3. Organization Learning	71
4. Overall Perceptions of Patient Safety and Quality	69
5. Staff Training	44
6. Owner/Managing Partner/Leadership Support for Patient Safety	31
7. Communication about Error	54
8. Communication Openness	52
9. Office Processes and Standardization	53
10. Work Pressure and Pace	21

Table 3. Composite average positive responses.

3.2. Data screening and pre-analysis

From an initial data set of 7299 respondents, it was removed 587 surveys with missing values and 2408 surveys with more than 2 answers on the option "not applicable," getting a final data set with 4304 surveys, exceeding the minimum necessary. The surveys with one answer in the option "not applicable" were replaced by the middle category in a five-point Likert scale.

3.3. Reliability analysis

Reliability analysis using Cronbach's α was performed on the 10 composites to ensure that individuals were responding consistently to items (**Table 4**). Considering Cronbach's α, all composites had values higher than 0.6, where composite 1 achieved the highest value and composite 9 the lowest. Analyzing AIIC coefficient, only composites 1 and 3 obtained values outside from the reference. In terms of global consistency, both coefficients lead to a good overall consistency.

Composite	No of items	Cronbach's α	AIIC
1. Teamwork	4	0.82	0.53
2. Patient Care Tracking/Follow Up	4	0.71	0.38
3. Organization Learning	3	0.79	0.56
4. Overall Perceptions of Patient Safety and Quality	4	0.69	0.38
5. Staff Training	3	0.69	0.43
6. Owner/Managing Partner/Leadership Support for Patient Safety	4	0.69	0.36
7. Communication about Error	4	0.75	0.43
8. Communication Openness	4	0.73	0.40
9. Office Processes and Standardization	4	0.63	0.31
10. Work Pressure and Pace	4	0.75	0.42
Total	38	0.92	0.24

Table 4. Internal consistency statistics.

3.4. Exploratory factor analysis

To examine whether a different structure would give a better fit to the data, an exploratory factor analysis was performed. To determine how many composites should be retained, it was obtained the path diagram in **Figure 1**, where a new structure is proposed. Eight composites were obtained with 37 items (item F6R was not considered since he had an eigenvalue lower than 0.4). Comparing this structure with the one proposed by MOSPSC, composites 1, 5, and 6 did not suffer any changes, composites 2 and 10 gained one item each, composite 4 lost 2 items, composite 8 gained one item and changed other, and composite 3 gained several items from composites 4, 7 and 9.

It was obtained the coefficients for internal consistency for the new proposed structure by EFA (**Table 5**). In a general way, it was obtained better internal consistency coefficients than with the original structure.

3.5. Confirmatory factor analysis

The fit of the data to the dimensional structure proposed in the original instrument was analyzed using structural equations models through confirmatory factor analysis (CFA). Correlations between composites are presented in **Table 6**, where it can be observed that there are

http://dx.doi.org/10.5772/intechopen.80035

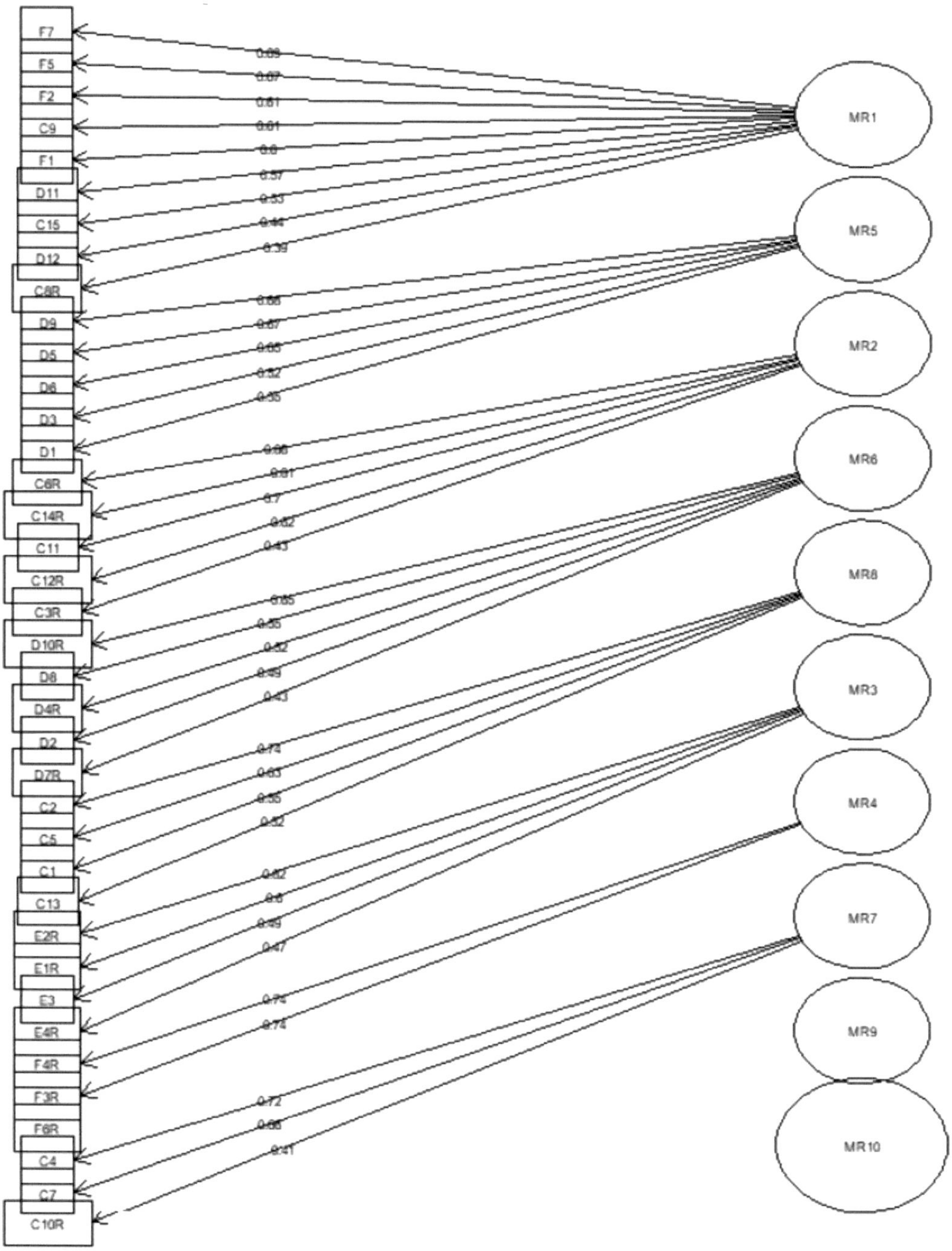

Figure 1. Path diagram of exploratory factor analysis. Rectangles represent items, circles represent factors (composites), and the values on the arrows are the eigenvalues.

Composite	No. of items	Cronbach's α	AIIC
1. Teamwork*	4	0.82	0.53
2. Patient Care Tracking/Follow Up + 8. Communication Openness (D1)	5	0.73	0.35
3. Organization Learning + 7. Communication about Error (D11, D12) + 9. Office Processes and Standardization (C9, C15) + 4. Overall Perceptions of Patient Safety and Quality (F2)	8	0.88	0.48
4. Overall Perceptions of Patient Safety and Quality [F2, F6R]	2	0.76	0.61
5. Staff Training*	3	0.69	0.43
6. Owner/Managing Partner/Leadership Support for Patient Safety*	4	0.69	0.36
8. Communication Openness [D1] + 7. Communication about Error (D7R) + 2. Patient Care Tracking/Follow Up (D8)	5	0.78	0.41
10. Work Pressure and Pace + 9. Office Processes and Standardization (C12R)	5	0.79	0.42
Total	38	0.92	0.243

*Composites who did not suffer any changes after EFA.
Curve brackets represent added items and rectangular brackets represent removed items from the composite.

Table 5. Internal consistency statistics after structure proposed by exploratory factor analysis.

	1	2	3	4	5	6	7	8	9	10
1	1									
2	0.495	1								
3	0.758	0.588	1							
4	0.591	0.533	0.859	1						
5	0.570	0.368	0.538	0.516	1					
6	0.405	0.302	0.520	0.515	0.549	1				
7	0.736	0.679	0.841	0.659	0.499	0.487	1			
8	0.788	0.622	0.773	0.648	0.498	0.463	0.893	1		
9	0.820	0.606	0.929	0.765	0.669	0.571	0.798	0.763	1	
10	0.147	0.117	0.191	0.270	0.357	0.326	0.230	0.153	0.530	1

Table 6. Correlations of the 10 composites.

high values between some composites. This will produce a nonpositive definite matrix of the covariances of the latent variables. In this sense, composite 9 was removed.

Figure 2 shows the relation of the individual items to the composites. The standardized path between coefficients shows the strength of these relations. A coefficient less than 0.1 indicates a low effect; coefficients around 0.3 indicate a medium effect, while large effects are suggested by coefficients higher or equal of 0.5. In this model, coefficients ranged between 0.45 and 0.87.

http://dx.doi.org/10.5772/intechopen.80035

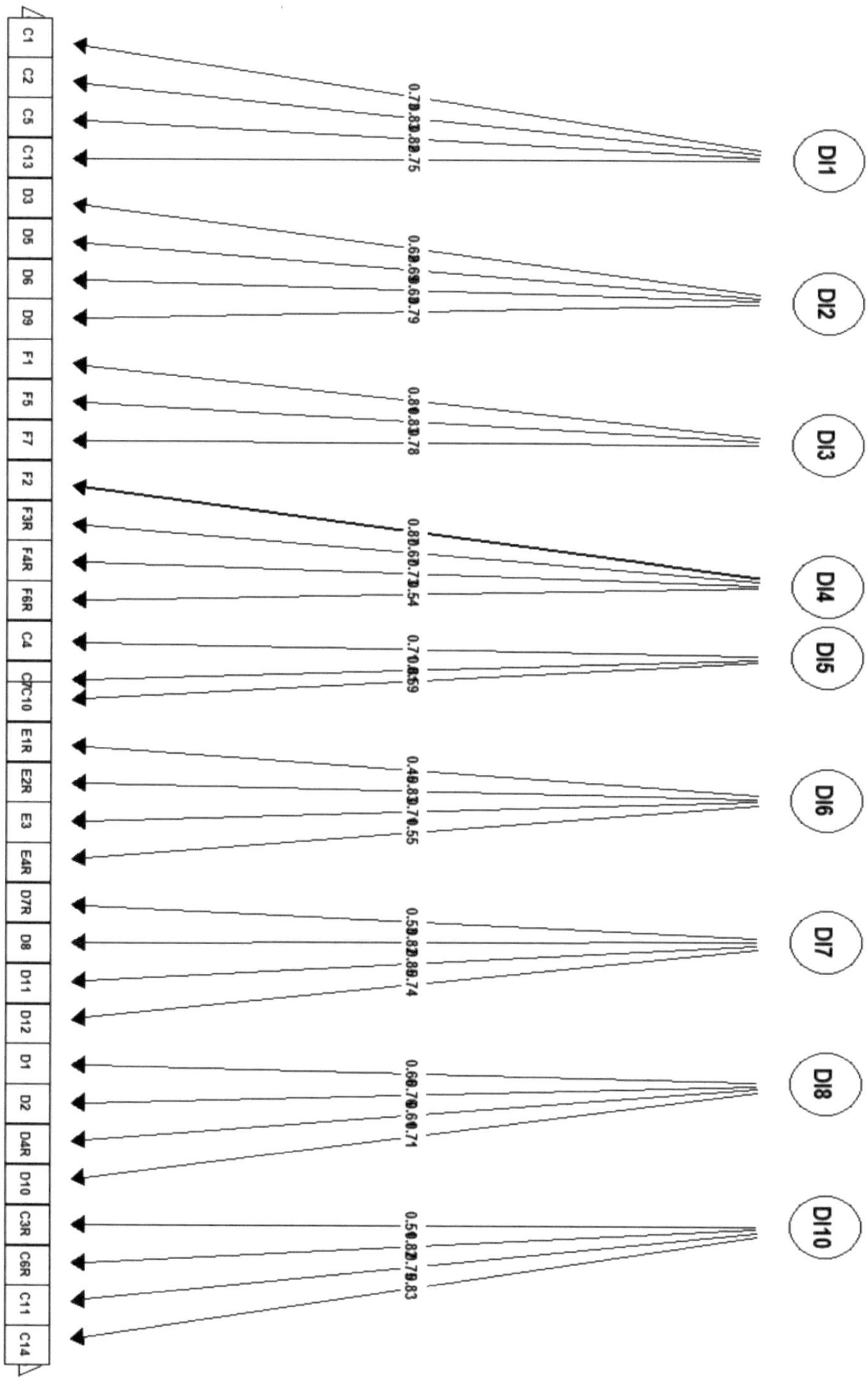

Figure 2. Confirmatory factor model where composite 9 was removed (34 items).

Table 7 shows the fit of the confirmatory factor analysis for the model proposed in **Figure 2**. The indices CFI and GFI showed a very good fit; RMSEA and TLI showed a good fit and PGFI a reasonable fit.

Goodness of fit indices	Values
CFI	0.98
TLI	0.97
PGFI	0.69
GFI	0.99
RMSEA	0.064 (p value < 0.001)

Table 7. Confirmatory factor analysis model fit indices.

It was also obtained a good overall internal consistency (Cronbach's $\alpha = 0.91$, AICC = 0.243).

Considering the model proposed by EFA (**Figure 1**), it was obtained the CFA model in **Figure 3**. In this model, coefficients ranged between 0.45 and 0.88.

The goodness-of-fit indices (**Table 8**) obtained for EFA model (**Figure 3**) are very similar to the ones obtained for the model proposed in **Figure 2**.

4. Discussion

We have described the results of a translation, an adaptation, and a validation and analyzed the reliability of the Medical Office Survey on Patient Safety Culture in Portuguese Primary Health Care. As far as we know, this is the first study on patient safety culture in primary health care in Portugal with this depth of analysis of the structure of the survey proposed by the Medical Office Survey.

The lowest positive scores were found in composites *Work Pressure and Pace, Owner/Managing Partner/Leadership Support for Patient Safety,* and *Staff Training.* The composites with highest scores were *Teamwork, Patient Care Tracking/Follow Up,* and *Organization Learning.*

The original survey had a good overall consistency, where the composite *Office Processes and Standardization* had the lowest values on internal consistency statistics and the composite *Teamwork* the highest. The exploratory factor analysis proposed a structure with eight composites, where just one item was removed, and several items were spread out by the others composites. Through confirmatory factor analysis, it was obtained another model structure where the composite *Office Processes and Standardization* was removed, leading to a survey with nine composites with 34 items. In terms of goodness of fit and internal consistency, there were no substance differences, both achieved good internal consistency and very good fit. It was decided to choose the structure proposed by CFA, since the differences in terms of structure to the original one are only by the removal of one composite, allowing comparison of the

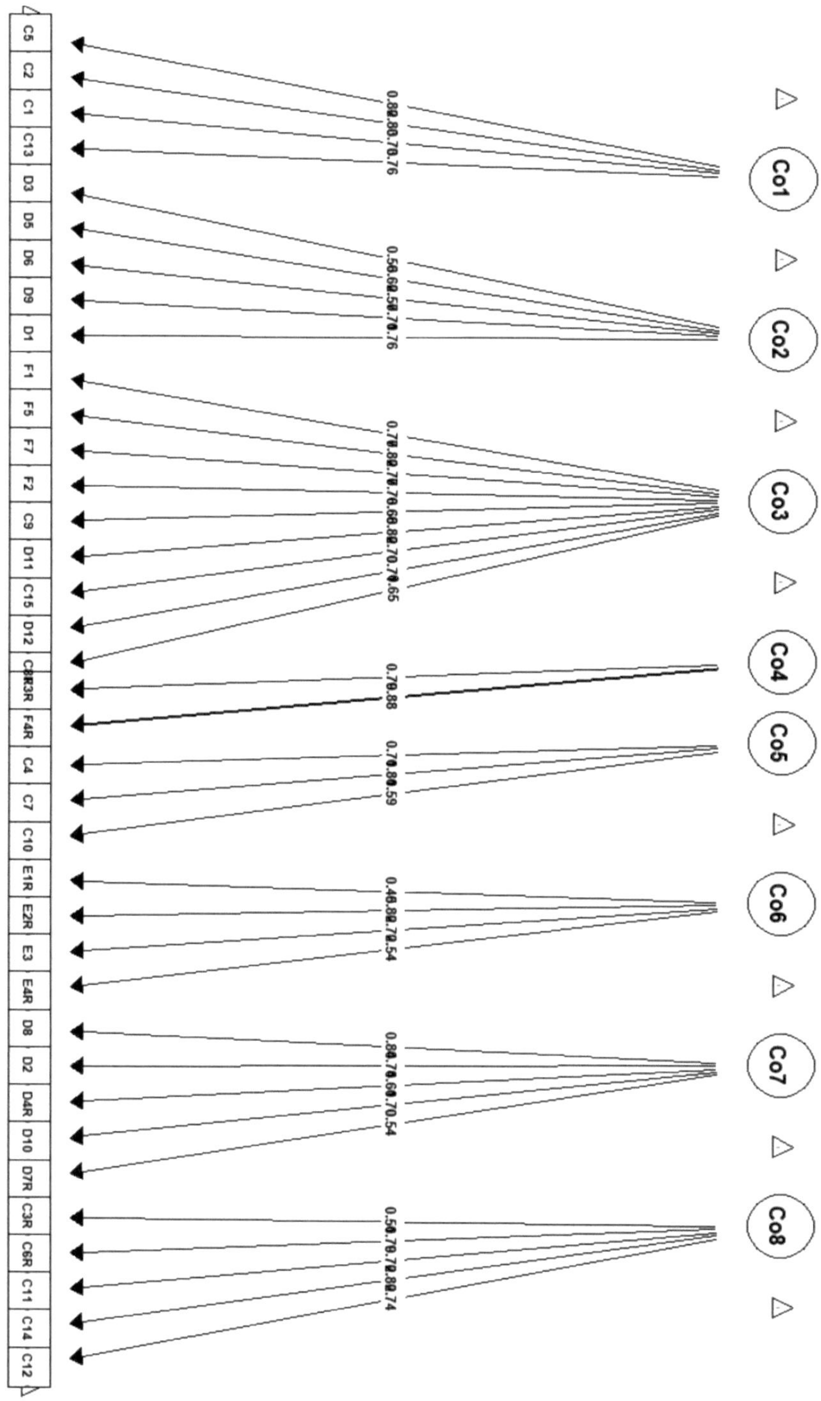

Figure 3. Confirmatory factor model for model proposed by EFA (37 items).

Goodness of fit indices	Values
CFI	0.98
TLI	0.97
PGFI	0.72
GFI	0.98
RMSEA	0.066 (p value < 0.001)

Table 8. Confirmatory factor analysis model fit indices for model proposed by EFA.

Portuguese results with the EUA results and other countries that get the same structure. Furthermore, this structure has a less number of items, getting a more parsimonious model.

A limitation of the study is the low response rate; however, it is not unusual for an open population study once it was Web-only administrated, although we have identified ways to publicize your survey and tracked response rates.

Another limitation of the study was the number of missing values. It reduced the representativeness of the sample and can therefore distort inferences about the population. In future studies, the results will be compared using imputation methods on missing values and the impact on the results will be evaluated.

A strength of this study is the statistical method used, particularly in exploratory factor analysis and confirmatory factor analysis, since they are the most appropriate to the data type of this study, where bias was reduced. The majority of the studies on the context of this study still use methods assuming that data are continuous.

As it is well known in Portugal, the Directory of Health has been doing patient safety culture assessment every 2 years since 2014, which allows all health units to enhance patient safety.

5. Conclusions

The Portuguese version of the MOSPSC resulted in nine composites with good reliability and construct validity, where the structure differs from the original by removing one composite. In further studies, it will be performed longitudinal studies to evaluate the impact of patient safety culture interventions on staff and patients.

Patient safety culture assessment is of a vital importance for all levels of care. In Portugal, we are caring out this assessment every 2 years, which allows institutions to identify patient safety culture status in primary care, and it is also seen as an intervention to raise staff awareness about patient safety issues and a mechanism to evaluate the impact of patient safety improvement initiatives. This assessment also allows primary care institutions to compare their patient safety culture survey results with others and is a way to track changes in patient safety culture over time.

http://dx.doi.org/10.5772/intechopen.80035

Acknowledgements

The authors would like to extend their gratitude to all staff that took time to complete the MOSPSC. This work is partially financed by national funds through FCT Fundação para a Ciência e a Tecnologia under the project UID/MAT/00006/2013 and by the Health and Technology Research Centre (H&TRC).

Conflict of interest

The authors declare that there are no conflicts of interest.

Ethical approval

The research complied with every one of the dilemmas concerned with ethics. The privacy and secrecy or anonymity of staff made certain.

Author details

Margarida Eiras[1]*, Ana Escoval[2] and Carina Silva[3]

*Address all correspondence to: margarida.eiras@estesl.ipl.pt

1 Escola Superior de Tecnologia da Saúde de Lisboa - Instituto Politécnico de Lisboa, Health and Technology Research Center (H&TRC), Portugal

2 National Public Health School of New University of Lisbon, CHLC, CISP, Portugal

3 Escola Superior de Tecnologia da Saúde de Lisboa - Instituto Politécnico de Lisboa, Statistics and Applications Center of the University of Lisbon, Health and Technology Research Center (H&TRC), Portugal

References

[1] Kohn LT, Corrigan JM, Donaldson MS. To Err Is Human: Building a Safer Health System. Washington, D.C.: National Academies Press; 2000

[2] Council of the European Union. Recommendation of 9 June 2009 on Patient Safety, including the Prevention and Control of Healthcare Associated Infections. OJEU. 2009;**C**(151):1-6

[3] National Patient Safety Agency: Seven steps to patient safety for primary care; 2006. Available at: http://www.aneezesmail.co.uk/PDF%20files/1791_7StepsToPrimaryCareIntroduction.pdf (accessed 25 may 2018)

[4] Vasconcelos PF, Arruda LP, Sousa Freire VEC, REFL C. Instruments for evaluation of safety culture in primary health care: integrative review of the literature. Public Health. 2018;**156**:147-151. DOI: 10.1016/j.puhe.2017.12.024

[5] Spencer R, Campbell SM. Tools for primary care patient safety: A narrative review. BMC Family Practice. 2014;**15**:166

[6] Verbakel N, Langelaan M, Verheij TJM, Wagner C, Zwart DLM. Improving patient safety culture in primary care: A systematic review. Journal of Patient Safety. 2016;**12**(3):152-158

[7] Stawicki SP, Firstenberg MS. Introductory Chapter: The Decades Long Quest Continues Toward Better, Safer Healthcare Systems, Vignettes in Patient Safety2017. DOI: 10.5772/intechopen.69354 Available from: https://www.intechopen.com/books/vignettes-in-patient-safety-volume-1/introductory-chapter-the-decades-long-quest-continues-toward-better-safer-healthcare-systems

[8] Sorra J, Gray L, Famolaro T, et al. AHRQ Medical Office Survey on Patient Safety Culture: User's Guide. (Prepared by Westat, under Contract No. HHSA290201300003C). AHRQ Publication No. 15(16)-0051-EF (Replaces 08(09)-0059). Rockville, MD: Agency for Healthcare Research and Quality; June 2016 http://www.ahrq.gov/professionals/quality-patientsafety/patientsafetyculture/medical-office/index.html

[9] Timm M, Rodrigues MC. Cross-cultural adaptation of safety culture tool for primary health care. Acta Paul Enferm. 2016;**29**(1):26-37. DOI: 10.1590/1982-0194201600005

[10] Parker D, Wensing M, Esmail A, Valderas JM. Measurement tools and process indicators of patient safety culture in primary care. A mixed methods study by the LINNEAUS collaboration on patient safety in primary care. European Journal of General Practice. 2015;**21**(Suppl 1):26-30. DOI: 10.3109/13814788.2015.1043732

[11] Dupie I, Nguyen Van Nhieu A: The medical office survey on patient safety culture MOSPSC: Opinions and views of EQuiP network general practitioners. http://equip.woncaeurope.org/8-working-groups/4-patient-safety

[12] Bland A, Altman G. Statistics notes: Cronbach's alpha. British Medical Journal. 1997;**314**:572

[13] Field A. Discovering Statistics Using SPSS for Windows. London: SAGE publications; 2000

[14] Clark LA, Watson D. Constructing validity: Basic issues in objective scale development. Psychological Assessment. 1995;**7**(3):309

[15] Baglin J. Improving your exploratory factor analysis for ordinal data: A demonstration using FACTOR. Practical Assessment, Research & Evaluation. 2014;**19**(5)

[16] Streiner DL. Figuring out factors: The use and misuse of factor analysis. The Canadian Journal of Psychiatry. 1994;**39**(3):135-140

[17] Revelle W. Psych: Procedures for Personality and Psychological Research. Northwestern University; 2018

[18] Fox J. The polycor Package: Polychoric and Polyserial Correlation. Version 0.7-1. 2016. Available at http://ftp.auckland.ac.nz/software/CRAN/ doc/packages/polycor.pdf (acessed 21 may 2018)

[19] Yves Rosseel lavaan. An R package for structural equation modeling. Journal of Statistical Software. 2012;**48**(2):1-36

Chapter 3

Communication in Surgery for Patient Safety

Daniel Kinyuru Ojuka, Lydia Okutoyi and
Frederick C. Otieno

Additional information is available at the end of the chapter

http://dx.doi.org/10.5772/intechopen.79740

Abstract

One of the cardinal pieces of the Hippocratic Oath is "do no harm"; yet, even in the very best of contexts, errors, at times fatal, do occur as was reported by the Institute of Medicine. Surgical procedures are known to cause the majority of serious adverse events. The Joint Commission report indicates that 60% of serious adverse events are caused by the lack of physician-patient communication. Some of the factors that make surgical processes prone to medical errors include the number of steps and people involved and the fact that the interventions intended for the healing are often in themselves invasive and can also complicate. The involvement of more than one discipline and individual requires communication that is clear, understandable, culturally sensitive, and contextually relevant. One of the center pieces of quality care is its patient-centeredness. This refers to providing service that is not only respectful but also responsive to individual patients involving them in the decisions, ensuring their values and preferences are taken into consideration. It also demands that the care giver provides the patients with relevant and understandable information to enable them in the decision-making and make informed choices.

Keywords: trust, vulnerability, communication, patient safety, quality of care, patient-centered, medical errors

1. Introduction

The doctor-patient communication can be said to have evolved over the centuries from that of paternalistic, to a collaboration that is more patient-centered [1]. In the history of medicine, the sociolinguistic structure of communication by doctors often maintained a style of high control, which Veatch in 1972 termed priestly style of doctor-patient relationship

[2, 3]. It has been noted that this high-handed or authoritarian style of communication leads to increased medical errors just as was observed in the aviation industry [4]. The Joint Commission sentinel data reports indicate that lack of communication is responsible for 60% of the adverse events [5]. A number of studies have highlighted the critical part communication plays both in the operating room and in the overall management of surgical patients [1, 3, 6]. A number of researches have highlighted the ways to communicate and the gaps in communication and why failure is more likely in surgical context [3]. This chapter aims to review the literature in communication from around the globe and to contextualize them into the developing world. This is because contexts differ, and similarly, infrastructure and culture may also differ.

2. Communicating with the surgical patient

Communicating with a surgical patient is unique in many ways since it will not only involve discussing the diagnosis and surgical management but also communicating with the team to care for the patient perioperatively. The central person and the team leader in these communications remains the surgeon. Communication can be defined as a process by which information is exchanged between individuals through a common system of symbols, signs, or behavior [7, 8]. This implies that at times, communications may not be effective not because the originator did not have the message but because something went wrong within the process of communication.

In this section, we will look at

- The communication processes
- Communication models
- Communicating with the patient
- Communicating with the team of care

2.1. The communication processes

In many books of communication, about 10 components in the communication process are emphasized. The steps include source, encoding, message, noise, media, receiver, decoding, receiver response, and feedback within a context.

The communication process involves the source, in this case, the surgeon or the trainee or the health care worker who wants to communicate with the receiver—the patient. Humans do not often share thoughts directly like computer gadgets. Therefore, the intended message ought to be encoded in ways that should be understandable by the receiver who would also need to decode it. Encoding is an active process of putting the thought into symbols which could be spoken words or unspoken symbols [9]. The receiver would assign meaning to symbols in another active process of decoding. The thoughts are encoded to a product called message, which is the intended thought you want the receiver to get [10]. The interface by which the source passes the encoded thoughts (message) to the receiver is media. This interface can get interference called noise that could be either external, internal, or semantic noise. External noise includes those issues that are outside of self that will distract from concentration. For example, reading while the television set is on. Internal noise includes thoughts, feeling, and conditions within an individual that could interfere with his or her concentration—for example, fatigue, hunger, and anger. Semantic noise includes the alternative ways in which the message could be decoded. Response could be action or inaction intended or not intended by the source's message; feedback then is what makes the source to acknowledge that communication was successful. Without feedback it would be difficult to know whether one has communicated successfully [8]. The context of communication and sitting arrangement matters a lot; the amount of light in a consultation room will help put the patient at ease. Culture as a component of context will be explored in the next section.

Awareness of the process and the pitfalls that could occur during communication is important. The physician-patient relationship has always been personal, so the media for better understanding would be face to face. The physician must set the environment that would enable successful communication including when family members are required—meaning many receivers. A key challenge is that surgery is a team work, and in any team work, communication is a core competency. Without clear, concise, brief, and timely "closed' communication, there would be confusion on goals, expectations, timing, and roles of each team player [11].

2.2. Communication models

Models of communication may help one understand what communication is and how it is performed:

i. Transmission model, where communication is a means of passing ideas from one person or organization to the other. Effectiveness is evaluated in terms of being able to manipulate others to the goal of the person communicating [6].

ii. Transactional model, where the source understands the receiver well enough to incorporate that knowledge in the encoding of the message such that the exact same words can be spoken to diverse audience with different meanings [6].

There are cultural modifications of these models. While the transmission model may appear to indicate superiority of the source, with a passive listener, some cultures tend to indicate the role of listener as critical in communication.

In Confucius culture, just as in cultures with high-power distance and are collectivistic, harmony and balance through proper behavior are highly regarded in such a way that:-.

a. A particular age determines how you communicate. In African culture, like Swahili, greetings differ with age—the young will use 'shikamo'. In Korean culture, terms of friendship differ with age—peers use 'chingu', younger on older people use 'adjussi/adjumoni' for male and female, respectively [8, 12].

b. A third party may be used to avoid confrontation with those respected. In African culture, this is seen in dowry negotiations [8].

c. Reciprocity is the basis of most relationships, which creates in a group deeper relationship where at times personal and business issues cross over, and is common in Confucius cultures [8].

In communication to the patient in a global village, and even within a country, one must be culturally sensitive. Cultural competency has been defined as the ability of providers and organizations to effectively deliver services that meet social, cultural, and linguistic needs of the patient.

The surgeons therefore must understand the culture and the language in which they practice and the meaning of both spoken and unspoken words in the culture to effectively develop a healing relationship with their patients. In order to heal, one must get into the world of the patient. This will enable them to empathize with them and help them understand their disease better in their own sociocultural context so as to help them overcome not only the disease but the illness as well [13].

In the intercultural communication, one must be sure to understand the different cultures and their emphasis; in medicine, one must understand the ethics practiced in different cultural contexts. Ethics then guides how one communicates. May and Sharratt identified four values in Western ethics namely autonomy, justice, responsibility, and care [14]. Menkiti identified African ethics to stress the well-being of the community and economic over political rights [15]. Other cultural values are more bent on the religion of the individual. Kales theory is that peace is the fundamental value interculturally; hence, ethical communicators ought to maintain that peace through respectful communication, not deliberately misleading, exercising the right to express one's self and identification with other cultures [16].

Several approaches for effective intercultural communication have been identified that include:

a. Business approach—maintenance of self, fostering relationship with the host, and promotion of correct perception of the environment [17]

b. Military approach [16]

- Self-respect—self-confidence
- Self-awareness—understanding how others would the other
- Empathy—viewing things through another person's eye
- Adaptability—ability to adjust to different environment
- Interaction—ability to effectively communicate with others
- Certainty—ability to accept contradictory situations
- Initiative—being open to new situations
- tolerance

c. Communication approach—respect for and tolerance of other cultures through four skill areas [16]:

   i. Personality strength—which involves knowing oneself, initiating a positive attitude, and being friendly through

      - self-concept—how one views themselves
      - self-disclosure—willingness to openly and appropriately reveal information about themselves
      - self-monitoring—using social information to control and modify self-presentation and expression
      - social relation—ability to reveal little anxiety about communication

   ii. Communication skills which involve being able to encode messages for people in diverse environments, interacting with them respectfully with flexibility [16].

      - Message skills—ability to understand and use language and feedback.
      - Behavioral flexibility-ability to select appropriate behavior in diverse situations
      - Interaction management—a person's other-oriented ability to initiate interactions, attentiveness, and responsiveness.
      - Social skills—involve empathy and identity maintenance where one is able to put themselves in the others person's stead—similar feelings and being able to give feedback that commensurate with the counterpart's identity.

   iii. Psychological adjustment—acclimatize to a new environment and cope with frustration such as stress and alienation (in ambiguous situations).

   iv. Cultural awareness.

2.3. Communicating with the patient

Communication between the physician and the patient can take the usual form of patient interview which comprises

i. information gathering and diagnostic formulation

ii. patient education

iii. shared-decision making

iv. delivering bad news

The outcome of the therapeutic encounter is dependent on effective communication; the communication begins with engaging the patient and involves being empathetic to the patient and family [18]. These two components are therefore the milieu that makes the four aspects mentioned above possible. The Institute for Healthcare Communication developed a communication for healthcare curriculum that mainly teaches 4-Es of communication, namely engage, empathize, educate, and enlist. In this section, we will consider more beginning with setting the environment right [19–21]. The Kalamazoo consensus added more that included building the doctor-patient relationship, opening the discussion, gathering information, understanding the patient's perspective, sharing information, reaching agreement on problems and plans, and providing closure [22].

2.3.1. Setting the stage

While the Institute for Healthcare Communication curriculum combines "engage" with "information gathering" for diagnostic purposes, "setting the stage for communication" should be treated differently [21]. The setting the stage for communication requires that the surgeon removes every distraction to help them focus on the patient, and it could have several components. It includes setting aside the phone, good posture that is upright and open, and a sitting position that is below the patient's eye level so as not to be threatening. There should be lighting in the consultation room. First impressions communicate many things, majorly the attitude of the individual. How we present ourselves to patients is critical in making the favorable first impression that can lead to a trusting partnership between the surgeon and the patient [23]. A smiling face, warm greeting that is coupled with introducing self and any other person in the room, and firm greeting or social touches will give an impression of openness and trustworthiness.

2.3.2. Information gathering

Having set the environment, the patient is engaged by eliciting the reason for the visit; this is usually done by open-ended questions. The patients should be allowed to tell their own story without interruption as one uses verbal and nonverbal cues to indicate active listening and keen interest in their words. Patient's story often should help in diagnostic formulation as well as their concerns, fears, and the impact of the disease in their life. They must be allowed to speak freely. The biomedical is the norm, but the patient should be looked at as the whole person.

The patient often has more than one concern; to avoid "doorknob syndrome", the provider needs to engage the patient to put all their agenda on the table [1]. This will help in prioritizing the agenda of the patient during this visit. Having stated the agenda, the surgeon can then clarify the agenda and summarize them as well. The physician, after listening to patient agenda, should agree with the patient on the agenda and also state what he intends to do [24]. Once the agenda is set, the patient is then allowed to tell the full story, and helped along using facilitative comments such as

- "tell me more"
- "Go on"

A good consultation skill is not just about history taking as learned in textbooks. A good history will include patient's ideas, concerns, expectations, and diagnosis. While it is important for the doctor to lay his agenda too, it should not be dominating the history taking. Listening and getting patient perspective is at the heart of good history taking. A true account of a patient's concern and how it has evolved over time requires practice, patience, understanding, and concentration. History is a sharing of experience between patient and doctor [25]. A consultation can allow a patient to unburden himself or herself.

2.3.3. *Empathize*

The ability to connect with the patient in a deep sense, pay attention keenly, and listen are central in clinical practice leading to patient trust in the physician and satisfaction of both the patient and the doctor. Empathy is the ability to understand the patient feelings, situation, and perspective and to communicate to the patient that one truly does understand. Done well, it helps promote diagnostic accuracy, therapeutic adherence, and patient satisfaction, while remaining time-efficient. Certain words facilitate empathy when used at the right time [26].

Empathy has cognitive, affective, and action components. The cognitive component requires the surgeon to "enter into" the perspective and experience of the patient by using verbal and nonverbal cues but does not lose own perspective or collapse clinical distance. Emotional component requires resonant feelings and the action required is the feedback. The surgeon could use statements such as "Let me see if I have this right" or "I want to be sure I understand what you mean." It helps give the patient a chance to correct but also connect and reinforces the bond between the surgeon and the patient [23].

Sympathy requires that the congruent feelings between the patient and the physician, while empathy does not. Even when patients are disagreeable, culpable, or unlikable, the surgeon can still empathize with them.

Barriers to empathy include time constraints, medical jargon, missing clues, and blocking behavior by the physician. Active listening means listening to and understanding the patient. The patients will give clues to their distress and the impact of their experience of illness; if we fail to acknowledge these clues, patients will repeat them that means prolonged patient visit and they will perceive us as "not listening, not caring, or in a rush." It is a good practice to have several empathic stems to use to allow one to fill in the blanks with the emotion or feelings witnessed [27]. The stems could be queries, responses, or clarifications. Such as:

i. Queries

- "Would you (or could you) tell me a little more about that?"
- "What has this been like for you?"
- "Is there anything else?"
- "Are you OK with that?"
- "Hmmmm"

ii. Clarifications

- "Let me see if I have this right."
- "I want to make sure I really understand what you're telling me. I am hearing that."
- "I don't want us to go further until I'm sure I've gotten it right."
- "When I'm done, if I've gone astray, I'd appreciate it if you would correct me. OK?"

iii. Responses

- "That sounds very difficult."
- "Sounds like ..."
- "That's great! I bet you're feeling pretty good about that."
- "I can imagine that this might feel ..."
- "Anyone in your situation would feel that way ..."
- "I can see that you are ..."

One serious issue why surgeons hardly empathize is the blocking behavior that could be done by offering advice or reassurance before the main problems have been identified, explaining away distress as normal, attending to physical aspects only, switching the topic, and "jollying" patients along [23, 26, 27].

2.3.3.1. Case scenario

The story: A 22-year-old girl was taken by her parents to see a general surgeon for breast lump. Her history did not indicate any risk but given the surgeon had just dealt with a 24-year-old lady with breast cancer, the surgeon preceded to perform mastectomy based on FNAC (core biopsy was then not readily available and was not the norm). The histological result of the mastectomy indicated fibroadenoma.

The patient's outcome: re-evaluation revealed that the history and examination did not align with FNAC and the surgeon should have asked for core biopsy. It is also possible that the pathologist mixed up results. The patient's parents filed suit against the original surgeon.

What went wrong? Cognitive bias and ignoring patient history and distraction from the previous patient made the surgeon to diagnose what was not there.

2.3.4. Patient education

One study comparing primary care physicians with surgeons showed that surgeons spend more time emphasizing patient education and counseling [28]. Given the complex intervention and the chances of complication, surgeons get involved in patient education so as to get informed consent. Unfortunately, much of the explanation is done through medical jargon, monolog without an attempt to seek the comprehension of the patient.

Other barriers to patient education are time pressure, language barrier, and limited health literacy [23, 27, 29].

Patient education is core to the two things for the surgeon namely, informed consent and shared decision-making, which are discussed in the next sub-section. The aim is to improve health literacy including knowledge and skills that are conducive for individual survival. It is performed in clinical setting and its goals are related to patient assessment, diagnosis, prognosis, evaluation, individual needs, and requirements related to interventions. The patient should receive education and training that is specific and appropriate to care, treatment, and service provided. It should be personalized to each patient depending on cultural differences, specific needs, and level of education [30].

At times, we try to force-feed the patients without assessing their understanding. Some of the strategies that have been suggested include "Ask me 3" from the National Patient Safety Foundation [31];

- What is my problem?
- What do I need to do?
- Why is it important for me to do this?

What is important is to break down the information in portions that the patient can understand, avoiding medical jargon, and using teach-back method to assess their comprehension. For example, instead of using 60%, use "6 out of 10".

The benefits of patient education include [30]

i. Patient assumes better responsibility for their own health care and ability to manage their own illness

ii. Provides opportunities to choose healthier lifestyle

iii. Increases patient satisfaction with their care, decreases providers risk of liability.

iv. Provides patient-centered care and as a result, patient's active involvement in their plan of care.

v. Increases adherence to treatment regimen, more efficient and cost-effective health systems.

vi. Ensures continuity of care, reduces complications related to illness.

vii. Maximizes individual independence with possible home care and plans.

2.3.5. Shared decision-making

This involves asking the patient to be involved in making the decision about his or her treatment. It involves discussing candidly all the options of treatment, including not treating at all, their merits, limitations, and complications. This, however, should be done respectfully and in an appropriate language and manner. It will also involve discussing patient values, preferences, and the best medical evidence that supports the treatment options in a language and respectful, empathic manner. The barrier would be patients' desire to be involved, physician knowledge of patient preference, and physician willing to explore patient concern and preferences [32].

The application of communication models is seen in decision-making in surgery where there are three ways namely, paternalistic model, informational model, and shared-decision making model. All these models have their merits and demerits and can actually be used by well-meaning surgeons. In the paternalistic model, the surgeon makes the decision and the patient accedes. This model best works in emergency situations. It leaves the patient uninformed, assumes that the patient preferences are aligned to the physicians, and leads to low adherence, less engagement during recovery and dissatisfaction with likelihood or litigation if untoward outcome occurs [33]. Informational model is where the physician will give only the information and let the patient decide. It assumes the patient is able to process and take into consideration their preferences. However, it has been noted that most patients are not able to process the information, and that given the emotions involved in sickness, some may even shut down because of information overload. Furthermore, often the physicians may give biased information. Shared decision involves giving information, hearing from patient and both parties participating to ensure understanding of patient preferences, and aligning the physician and patient. It also involves assessing patient judgment [34].

The traditional style of paternalistic communication may not welcome patient's input and the patient may also fear being labeled as a 'difficult' patient. But the reward will be that when patients understand their diagnosis, the implication of treatment, and possible outcomes, they would own the process and would adhere to treatment protocols [33]. Many other things could affect adherence and include social support, financial concern, and communication with the doctor. It may therefore call for exploring the social support and enlisting family or other important people in their lives. In some cultures, such as Africa, some of the decisions will have to be family-based.

Several factors may influence patient choice, including information from physician, from family, from internet, and other media sources. The physician can also be influenced by the industry, recommendation made previously that may not be useful for the current illness or articles read with evidence. Certain patient personalities may also be barriers to shared decision-making; there are patients who will leave the decision to the physician—they prefer minimal information, others may prefer information only. The physician may also fail to provide a conducive environment when they discount patient preferences and concerns. Other barriers include time constraint and physician attitude—some may feel shared decision-making is not necessary. The physician must ensure the information given is of right quality (understood) and quantity (not overwhelming) [32].

The patient perspective while making decisions may be fourfold. They may feel the decision is obvious and can be done immediately or feel overwhelmed and defer it to someone else or just require time to process and they may require more information to make the decision. The surgeon must allow the patient time and space to go through the motions. Though it may take time, once shared decision is made, the process will be long and compliance will be total [32].

2.3.5.1. *Case scenario*

The story:

Ms. Rono presented to a health clinic for assessment for a job. When the physicians perform examination, he finds a 1 cm x 1 cm lump on the right upper outer quadrant. A mammogram indicates it is BIRAD 4c. He refers the patient to Dr. Otieno, the breast surgeon. Dr. Otieno confirms the finding and begins talking to Ms. Rono, taking history and performing physical examination. Dr. Otieno gets to know Ms. Rono's preference, interest, and life plans. Dr. Otieno incorporates this knowledge into subsequent discussions about choices for medical treatment.

Although it may seem a straightforward decision of biopsy on a palpable lump, Dr. Otieno needs to consider age, physical condition, and whether she would be able to undergo the treatment based on the results of the biopsy. Equally important would be whether Ms. Rono would want any treatment if the biopsy revealed a malignancy.

The process should proceed in this manner.

Discuss the risks associated with biopsy. Dr. Otieno should discuss the risk of biopsy itself that includes infection, bleeding, and cosmetic consequences of the scar. He should ask the patient questions about her concern and preferences that may arise from her own research or information from family, friends, and media. Address these concerns at this time.

Determine whether the patient is competent to make decisions. This is often determined based on the ability of the patient to understand the information and situation awareness, weigh options, and make and communicate their choice. For Ms. Rono, this includes her circumstances of coming for check up for a job but now has a new diagnosis. If Ms. Rono is not competent, then Dr. Otieno should seek out her durable attorney and discuss with her. The capacity to comprehend is assessed by using teach-back method.

The patient's outcome:

Ms. Rono and Dr. Otieno make shared decisions to proceed with the biopsy. The biopsy turns out to be positive for breast malignancy.

Dr. Otieno's subsequent talks with Ms. Rono require being comprehensive and includes patient's preferences and concerns. He should give her options of treatment without surpassing her capacity to understand. The patient potential circumstances should be considered as she is offered breast conserving surgery (BSCS) versus mastectomy. Can the patient access and afford radiation after the BCS?

Most patients take time to make a decision and will take more than one visit. The informed consent and shared decision-making process take time as patient looks for more information and do further consultation of family and friends. Decision aids such as pamphlets will be important because she can review the information when she feels she is not under stress.

The informed consent should be performed by the person doing the procedure or understands the procedure. It should include indications for procedure, steps of the procedure, potential complications, benefits of the procedure, options and complications of the alternative procedures, and risk of not doing anything. Finally, the patient competence and understanding should be assessed. The core principles of informed consent are that it is not the paper that matters but the process of involving the patient [33, 34]. It is therefore an opportunity to help the patient come to shared decision rather than obligation for the surgeon. It is very helpful as a first step of disclosure should something go wrong and applies to all medical treatment.

Surgeons should be transparent and truthful about their experience and the data that are available when a patient asks for risk of complications of procedures without being too detailed in order to help patients in decision-making about their care. The physician should help the patient interpret data that is available in broad terms as was suggested above [32].

Ms. Rono is choosing whether to undergo mastectomy, or BCS, then radiation. Dr. Otieno should understand Ms. Rono's preferences. It is possible that Ms. Rono is most interested in pursuing the treatment that is likely to leave her with a breast rather than understanding slight differences in 5-year recurrence rates. Dr. Otieno needs to elicit these priorities during the conversation about surgical options. At the same time, if Dr. Otieno is excited about a new surgical modality, like BCS, he needs to be truthful about what the data say and his own experience with the procedure.

2.3.6. Delivering bad news

The "news" to the patient after clinical assessment or investigation is potentially bad news. Buckman defines bad news as "any information which adversely and seriously affects an individual's view of his or her future" [35]. However, it is the patient who knows what they consider as bad news. The impact of bad news can only be determined after the recipient's expectations and understanding are known. Ms. Rono's biopsy results could cause her shock given she did not go with the knowledge of the lump to the doctor.

Sharing of bad news can be difficult for the doctor based on certain factors such as fear of being blamed for the bad news, fear of arousing strong emotions or causing pain, uneasiness with their inability to make the disease go away or to answer all the patient's questions, difficulty in facing death, and discomfort arising from the fact that they simply do not know how to carry out the task well [35].

Sharing bad news is frequent and stressful but it is what needs to be done because patients require knowing the truth about their diagnosis and prognosis. This needs to be handled sensitively and sincerely. The practice of deception cannot instantly be remedied by a new routine of insensitive truth telling [36]. The way bad news is discussed can affect the patient's understanding of information, satisfaction with medical care, level of hopefulness, and subsequent psychological adjustment [35]. As much as many patients desire accurate information to help them make important quality-of-life decisions, some may find it threatening and may get into denial or minimizing the significance of the information while continuing with care.

The goal of breaking bad news is fourfold, firstly, to gather information on what the patients know, their readiness, and their expectations; secondly, to provide appropriate information according to patient needs, expectation, and desires; thirdly, to support the patient by reducing emotional impact and isolation experienced by the patient; and finally, to formulate treatment plan in shared decision model.

This can be done in six steps [36].

a. Setting up

  i. The patient and relatives if present require a setting that would be private and if possible have tissues in case patient is upset.

  ii. It is important that the patients have relatives or friends comfortable to accompany them during these discussions.

  iii. Posture and sitting arrangement should be ones that help calm the patient and makes them relax.

  iv. Eye contact, holding the patient's hand, or any social touch may help make connection with the patient.

  v. Ensure there are no possible interruptions within the time.

b. Assessing patient perception.

Before discussing medical findings, clinical or investigations, the clinician should use open-ended questions to create a reasonably accurate picture of how the patients perceive their medical situation.

  i. "What have you been told about your situations so far?"

  ii. "What is your understanding of the reason we did the mammogram?"

This information can then be used to correct any misinformation and contextualize the bad news to the patient's understanding. It may also help to find out if the patient is in denial either through wishful thinking or omission of essential but unfavorable details or unrealistic expectations.

c. Obtaining patient invitation.

Although most patients desire full information about their diagnosis and prognosis, some may not. Expressing desire for the information may place the surgeon at ease, and shunning information may indicate a coping mechanism and may be a sign of severity of illness. The surgeon may prepare the patient at the time of ordering the test by asking

  i. "How would you like me to give the information about the test results?"

  ii. "Would you like me to give you all the information or sketch out the results and spend more time in planning the treatment?"

In case they do not want details, the surgeon can offer to answer any question they may have in future.

d. Giving patient information

Words that express some form of warning before the bad news is given may prepare the patient, lessen the shock, and help in processing the information. This may be expression such as

i. "Unfortunately, I have some bad news to tell you"

ii. "I am sorry to tell you that ..."

Give medical fact by knowing the level of understanding and using correct vocabulary. Avoid excessive bluntness that may leave the patient isolated and later angry with a tendency to blame the surgeon-such language as—"your cancer is very bad and if not treated immediately you are going to die". Give information in small portion, check patient understanding at every step, and finally, even if prognosis is poor, avoid using phrases that discourage such as 'there is nothing we can do for you', because the goal of pain and symptom relief is still options.

e. Being empathetic

This has been addressed above, but for emphasis, patient emotional reactions may vary from silence to disbelief, crying, denial, or anger. The physician can offer support by giving empathic response in four steps.

i. Take the cues that may include sadness, silence, or crying

ii. Confirm the emotions with the patient by open questions

iii. Confirm the reason for emotion, mostly connected with bad news

iv. Let the patient know you understand why they could be sad.

f. Strategy and summary

A clear plan and strategy may make the patient less anxious and more certain. However, the treatment options should be discussed with the patient who is 'available' emotionally. If the physician continues, it may appear like the physician's preferences are more important than patients. Shared decision-making model engenders shared responsibility and reduces sense of failure when treatment is not successful. Ensuring the patient has understood, documenting the finding, and recording all that is said and done are important.

3. Communicating with the team of care

Surgery is a complex procedure that involves the patient, surgeon, anesthesiologist, nurses, technician, and relatives and for complete care of patient: nutritionist, physiotherapist, internist, radiologist, pathologist, radiotherapy experts, and many more. This complexity begins from the time the patient is admitted from outpatient, through ward, operating room, postoperative acute room, and back to the ward and follow up. It is this complexity that could lead to medical error as a result of miscommunication. The Agency for Healthcare Research and Quality (AHRQ) developed tools for communication among the surgical team that aligns the surgical care well. This is called TeamSTEPPS [37].

The tool begins with at the structure of communication. The structure is called multi-team system for patient care. Team is defined as two or more people who interact dynamically, interdependently, and adaptively towards a common and valued goal, have specific roles or functions, and have a time-limited membership [37]. The core team is a group of care providers with the closest contact with the patient. They work interdependently to manage patients from point of assessment to disposition. In the case scenario of Ms. Rono, this would include Dr. Otieno, surgical resident, intern, and the ward nurse. Contingency team is a time-limited team formed for emergent or specific events and composed of members from various teams. This will be the operating room team or the code blue team: a team comprising members are responsible for managing the operational environment that supports the core team. Ancillary Services provide direct, task-specific, and time-limited care to patients while also support services provide indirect service-focused tasks which help to facilitate the optimal health care experience for patients and their families. This includes nutritionist, physiotherapist, and social workers [37].

The role of administrators is to establish and communicate vision, develop policies, and set expectations for staff related to teamwork, support and encourage staff during implementation and culture change, hold teams accountable for team performance, and define the culture of the organization. The patient is as the apex of the pyramid, indicating every team is involved in taking care of the patient (**Figure 1**).

The team structure is important because it identifies individuals among which information must be communicated, designates leaders, and mutual support is sought. In a complex scenario such as this, between-team communication and within-team communication about tasks and processes are important. Effectiveness of teams can be sabotaged by factors that are described by Lencioni in his book: The Five Dysfunctions of a Team. This includes inattention to results, avoidance of accountability, lack of commitment, fear of conflict, and absence of trust [38]. Therefore, team leadership with concomitant effective communication is key to patient safety in such context.

In this complexity, effective communication serves as the coordinating mechanism for the teamwork and is the lifeline of a well-functioning team. The skills to communicate effectively are essential for patient safety and are the mode by which most of the tools for TeamSTEPPS are executed. The sentinel event data reported by the Joint Commission between 1995 and 2005 indicate that ineffective communication was the root cause of 66% of the errors reported. The data from 2010 to 2013 indicate that ineffective communication remain among the top three causes of sentinel events [5].

Failure of communication within the team or department leads to failure to share information with the team, failure to request information from others, or direct information to a particular member of the team and also failure to include patients and their families in communication involving their care. This will be indicated by poor documentation, that is not timed,

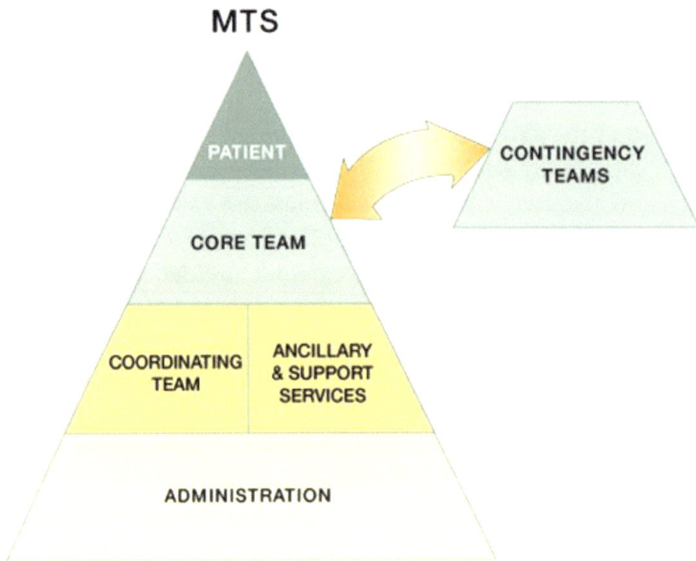

Figure 1. Multiple team systems.

nonspecific, and incomplete and failure to seek input from the patient. In case of automated systems, it will also lead to inconsistencies in the utilization of the system [37].

Effective communication is complete, clear, timely, and brief. Complete means communicating essential information without giving details that may cause confusion and letting the receiver have an opportunity for clarification. Clear information is one that uses plain language that can be understood by patients and relatives or standard terminologies understandable to every healthcare provider. Brief means being concise and to the point and timely implies being dependable to offer and seek information, without delays in relaying or getting information that could compromise patient care, recheck, and validate information [37].

Challenges to effective communication include language barriers, distractions such emergency, distance, and personalities that are difficult to communicate with, heavy workload and varying communication styles, and disagreement which may disrupt flow of information. Lack of verification and acknowledgement of received information and transitions in care of patient can lead to communication breakdown [37].

3.1. Case scenario

Ms. Rono, having been investigated, is now admitted for breast conserving surgery. However, the surgeon who saw her at outpatient is called for an emergency. The trainee assumes that mastectomy would be better without reference to patient or Dr. Otieno, so they perform mastectomy instead of breast conserving surgery.

This scenario is common where there is no clear and effective communication. A number of tools have been developed for communication in varying scenarios. Effective teams are led by

http://dx.doi.org/10.5772/intechopen.79740

leaders who model communication to achieve team cohesiveness and effectiveness. This leads to better outcomes to the patient's and surgeon's satisfaction. For communication within and between teams to be effective, the leadership must have a style that facilitates it. A surgeon may have a disruptive style of communication that puts the patient at risk of mistakes during procedures. It interferes with cohesiveness and minimizes the chances of juniors raising concerns because the environment is not conducive. There are tools that have been developed to aid teams be effective in their communication, maintain their cohesiveness, and have clear explicit messages understood and accepted by all members of the team. These tools include ISBAR, call-outs, handoffs, and check-backs.

ISBAR is a tool that was developed for healthcare workers to communicate about a patient's condition. It helps organize one's thoughts to communicate clearly and completely [37].

I-Introduce yourself.

S-Situation that has made you call.

B-Background of the patient condition and current status.

A-assessment that has led to the concern.

R-Recommendation for the condition.

3.2. Case scenario

It is post-mastectomy day one for Ms. Rono; her drainage tube is not working well and the mastectomy site is full because of hematoma/seroma. The patient is in pain. The nurse is notified and so she decides to escalate the problem to the surgeon. She would identify herself by her name and state that Ms. Rono has a postmastectomy hematoma; she is a patient who had right sided mastectomy the day before, and currently her drain is not working well. She has examined and found the mastectomy site to be swollen and warm and suggests that another drain would help.

While doing this, the nurse and the doctor can use check-back or closed-loop systems that ensure that the message passed by the nurse is repeated to her by Dr. Otieno and she acknowledges and ascertains the message being passed; this helps in verification of the message. In situation where, for example, Ms. Rono has bled a lot and requires the resuscitation team, the nurse would have to use call-out, which means sending the message to all the members of the team at once. It is a method of sending critical information during an emergent event. The information is used to prepare the team members to anticipate what the situation is and how to act. Usually the team leader may distribute tasks that need to be performed to specific members; the check-back confirms that the team member has received and understood the message [37].

Most of the hospital staff works in shifts, and it has been noted that most of the adverse events occur during this change-over period. If the nurse in the morning had noticed the hematoma and because of distraction had not called and fails to notify his or her colleagues in the next shift, that patient may not be attended to until she requires resuscitation, if the bleeding remains active. To avoid such events, there is a tool used for handoffs, which aims to provide accurate information about a patient's care, treatment and services, current condition, and any recent or anticipated changes. The information communicated during a handoff must be accurate to meet patient safety goals [37].

Handoff needs to include transfer of both accountability and responsibility, the person assuming responsibility must be aware of what they are assuming, and the person handing over is responsible until both parties are aware of the transfer. It is the responsibility of the person transferring responsibility to clear up any uncertainty and ambiguity. While it is important to write and document the issues about the patients, it is reckless to assume that the person obtaining responsibility will read or understand written or nonverbal communication. Use of checkbacks also does help because it is until the receiver has acknowledged that the handoff is understood and accepted that the responsibility is relinquished. It may also be an opportunity to review the patient with new thoughts both for quality and safety, review the certainty of diagnosis, and patient response to treatment, and recent changes either in plans or response and other contingencies can be reviewed. Handoffs ensure continuity of care for the patient and hence increase chances of better outcome for the patient [37].

One of the tools used is I PASS the BATON mnemonic, which means

- I—The person handing over introduces themselves
- P—They then give a summary of the patient illness including name, identifiers, age, sex, and location.
- A—They detail the assessment, like chief complaint, vital signs, symptoms, and diagnosis
- S—The situation the patient is in currently including code status, level of uncertainty, recent changes, and response to treatment.
- S—Safety concerns—recent lab values and reports of concern, socio-economic factors, alerts, and allergies
- Background—Comorbidities, previous episodes, current medications, and family history
- Action—What actions were taken or are required? Provide brief rationale for the actions
- Timing—Level of urgency and explicit timing and prioritization of actions
- Ownership—Who is responsible (nurse/doctor/team)? Includes patient/family responsibilities
- Next—What will happen next? Anticipated changes? What is the plan? Are there contingency plans.

It is important for the person taking over to verbally question, confirm, and challenge the assumptions of those who take care of the patient at this point. The clinical team leadership for the surgical patient is always the surgeon. The surgeon is therefore expected to model appropriate behavior, share information proactively, defer to expertise or delegate as appropriate, use resources appropriately, provide feedback and coach those he leads, assist team members to manage conflicts, and always act in patient's interest [37].

One of the most effective communication tools that surgical teams have ever used that have reduced medical errors in operative room is the WHO operative checklist. It helps the team of the surgeon, anesthesia, scrub nurse, circulating nurse, and technicians communicate smoothly. Surgical team leaders share information proactively with their teams, using components of the safe surgical checklist including briefings, huddles, and debriefings. They will initiate and ensure that the time-outs are run. They can delegate or defer to experts and currently there is enough information to say that surgical teams who do not use surgical checklist endanger the patient. When it was introduced, the recorded reduction in mortality was 47% and reduction in complication was 35%. Surgical teams who use these skills capture errors before they can cause patient harm and it is the responsibility of the surgeon to ensure that all the elements of the checklist are performed as intended [39–41].

The entire surgical team introduce themselves and their roles before the incision and agree on the surgical procedure, surgical site and preoperative prophylaxis. During the first briefing, the surgeon shares the surgical plan, possible difficulties, expected duration, anticipated blood loss, and implants or equipment needed. The anesthesiologists also share their plan, their airway concerns including equipment. The nursing team shares sterility of equipment issues and other concerns they may have. Debriefing is sign out part that ensures the counts are fine, records are kept of the procedure, specimen is labeled, and a review of what was done in terms of roles, what went well, what should we change, and what can improve. Any error avoided, did we ask or offer assistance and was situation awareness maintained, was communication clear [40].

Within the checklist is included one of the tools that not only help with safety but also quality improvement and that are debriefing (**Table 1**). It should be done by the clinical team leader when everyone is still in the room, after sponge count, specimen is labeled, and procedure identification is done. The surgeon should facilitate the discussion by asking some of the questions above; they could also recap the situation, background, nay key event that occurs and summarize the lessons learnt.

Given the nature of surgery is that of teamwork, it is inevitable that conflict will arise because of differences in clinical knowledge, work approaches, values, opinions, or personality. Conflict resolution is key to delivering safe quality surgical care. Skills for resolving conflict will enhance team effectiveness and improve their outcomes. An effective leader will not allow interpersonal or irrelevant issues to negatively affect the team. They should not avoid but acknowledge and assist the team members to manage conflict with two challenges—CUS and DESC [37].

DESC challenge is a constructive approach of managing and resolving conflict that involves describing the specific situation, expressing your concern about the action, and suggesting alternatives while stating the consequences of the actions. The effectiveness of this method could be maximized by having timely discussion, in a private place, framing the problem in one's own experience and working for the right of the patient, using "I", avoiding blame games, focus on what is right not on who is right, critiquing, and not criticizing [37].

CUS challenge is that for being concerned or need clarity, I am uncomfortable, this is safety issues (I am scared STOP!). These two challenges are useful in raising concern about safety [37].

Before anesthesia	Before skin incision	Before patient leaves operating room
Sign in	Time out	Sign out
Patient has confirmed • Identity • Site • Procedure • Consent	Confirm all team members have introduced themselves by name and role	Nurse verbally confirms with the team: The name of the procedure recorded the instrument, sponge and needle counts are correct (or not applicable) How specimen is labeled (Including patient name).
Site marked/not applicable	Surgeon, anesthesia professional and nurse verbally confirm • Patient • Site • Procedure	Whether there are any equipment problems to be addressed.
Anesthesia check list completed Pulse oximeter on patient and functioning	Anticipated critical events • Surgeon reviews: what are the critical or unexpected steps, operative duration, and anticipated blood loss. Anesthesia team: Are there any patient-specific concerns • Nursing team reviews: Has sterility (including indicator results) been confirmed? Are there equipment issues or concerns?	Surgeon, anesthesia professional and nurse review the key concerns for recovery and management of this patient (Debrief). • *Communication clear?* • *Roles and responsibilities understood?* • *Situation awareness maintained?* • *Workload distribution?* • *Did we ask for or offer assistance?* • *Were errors made or avoided?* • *What went well, what should change, what can improve?*
Does the patient have • Known allergies: Yes/No • Difficult airway/aspiration risk No/Yes, and equipment assistance available • Risk of >500 ml of blood loss (7 ml/Kg for children) No/Yes and adequate intravenous access and fluid available	Has antibiotic prophylaxis been given within the last 60 minutes? Yes/Not applicable Is essential imaging displayed Yes/Not applicable.	

Table 1. WHO safety checklist.

Everyone in the team should be made aware that it is their responsibility to assertively raise their voice at least two times to ensure they are heard, that the member being challenged must acknowledge, and that if the outcome is not acceptable, a stronger action should be taken with the supervisor and that there should be stop the line in issues about safety including cessation of the process. While conflicts are common, that about 40% of the leader's time is spend on this, solving is critical to becoming productive and increase possibility of satisfaction of the physician and patient [37].

There are other ways of managing conflict that has not been found to improve patient outcomes. These include compromise where both parties settle for less, avoidance where the issue is sidestepped or ignored altogether, accommodation or deference where the focus on preserving the relationship and not the patient interest override, or dominance where the higher status member wins or whoever yells the loudest. When the surgeon words belittle or intimidate members, it inhibits willingness to speak up and hence the surgeon must be willing to listen, follow ad model effective communication, and be the role model [37].

4. Conclusion

For medicine to be healing, communication with patient and other healthcare workers must be effective and efficient. The traditional models of communications in principle and theory are changing to include consideration for the global nature of the practice of medicine. New models and tools for better communication with colleagues, patients, and their relatives have been developed. Research has indicated that those who use these tools consistently have not only gained clarity in their communication but they improve physician-patient relationship and outcomes as well. Cultural considerations and modifications of models to fit international communication have led to the need of cultural competency in clinical practice. All these efforts are employed to ensure that consideration is given to the patient and outcomes in whatever context they may be. In communication, there can be misunderstanding; these must be solved speedily and in a way that is respectful to both party's perspectives so that the main interest remains the good of the patient.

Acknowledgements

I acknowledge the contribution of my colleagues, Dr. Okutoyi and Prof Otieno.

Conflict of interest

None to declare.

Author details

Daniel Kinyuru Ojuka[1]*, Lydia Okutoyi[2] and Frederick C. Otieno[3]

*Address all correspondence to: danielojuka@gmail.com

1 Department of Surgery, University of Nairobi, Nairobi, Kenya

2 Department of Quality and Patient Safety, Kenyatta National Hospital, Kenya

3 School of Medicine, University of Nairobi, Kenya

References

[1] Ha JF, Longnecker N. Doctor-patient communication: A review. The Ochsner Journal. 2010;**10**(1):38-43

[2] Veatch RM. Models for ethical medicine in a revolutionary age. The Hastings Center Report. 1972:5-7. DOI: 10.2307/3560825

[3] Francis V, Korsch BM, Morris MJ. Gaps in doctor-patient communication: Patients' response to medical advice. The New England Journal of Medicine. 1969;**280**(10):535-540. DOI: 10.1056/NEJM196903062801004

[4] Hull L, Arora S, Aggarwal R, Darzi A, Vincent C, Sevdalis N. The impact of nontechnical skills on technical performance in surgery: A systematic review. Journal of the American College of Surgeons. 2012;**214**(2):214-230. DOI: 10.1016/j.jamcollsurg.2011.10.016

[5] Commission J. Sentinel Event Data: Root Causes by Event Type. Oakbrook Terrace IL; 2015

[6] Berlo DK. The Process of Communication: An Introduction to Theory and Practice. New York:Holt, Rinehart and Winston; 1960

[7] Communication | Definition of Communication by Merriam-Webster [Internet]. Available from: https://www.merriam-webster.com/dictionary/communication [Accessed: April 29, 2018]

[8] Communication as an Element of Culture | Cross Cultural Communication | Confucianism [Internet]. Scribd. Available from: https://www.scribd.com/document/78950339/Communication-as-an-Element-of-Culture [Accessed: June 2, 2018]

[9] Tobin JL, Dobard RG. Hidden in Plain View: A Secret Story of Quilts and the Underground Railroad. New York: Random House Inc, Anchor; 1999

[10] DeVito JA. The Communication Handbook: A Dictionary. New York: Harper & Row; 1986

[11] Yule S, Flin R, Paterson-Brown S, Maran N. Non-technical skills for surgeons in the operating room: A review of the literature. Surgery. 2006;**139**(2):140-149. DOI: 10.1016/j.surg.2005.06.017

[12] Kopytoff I. Ancestors as elders in Africa. Africa. 1971;**41**(02):129-142. DOI: 10.2307/1159423

[13] Hampden-Turner CM, Trompenaars F. Building Cross-Cultural Competence: How to Create Wealth from Conflicting Values. Yale; Yale University Press; 2008. ISBN 9780300084979. Available from: https://books.google.co.ke/books?id=SEZnmAEACAAJ

[14] May L, Sharratt SC. Applied Ethics: A Multicultural Approach. Upper Saddle River, New Jersey: Prentice Hall; 1994. 582 p

[15] Communitarianism in African Thought—Menkiti On Communitarianism—Person, Personhood, Individual, and Community—JRank Articles [Internet]. Available from: http://science.jrank.org/pages/8771/Communitarianism-in-African-Thought-Menkiti-on-Communitarianism.html [Accessed: June 2, 2018]

[16] Jandt FE. An Introduction to Intercultural Communication: Identities in a Global Community. Thousand Oaks, California: Sage Publications Inc; 2017

[17] Poole M. Human Resource Management: Critical Perspectives on Business and Management. Thames, Oxfordshire United Kingdom, Routledge Taylor & Francis; 1999. 424 p

[18] Novack DH. Therapeutic aspects of the clinical encounter. In: The Medical Interview (Part of Frontiers of Primary care by Mack Lipkin, Jr The medical interview/Mack Lipkin, Jr., Samuel M. Putnam, Aaron Lazare. p. cm. Includes bibliographical references and index. Springer; 1995. pp. 32-49. ISBN-13: 978-1-4612-7559-6. DOI: 10.1007/978-1-4612-2488-4 e-ISBN-13: 978-1-4612-2488-4). DOI: 10.1007/978-1-4612-2488-4_3

[19] Haig KM, Sutton S, Whittington J. SBAR: A shared mental model for improving communication between clinicians. Joint Commission Journal on Quality and Patient Safety. 2006;**32**(3):167-175. DOI: 10.1016/S1553-7250(06)32022-3

[20] Pronovost P, Berenholtz S, Dorman T, Lipsett PA, Simmonds T, Haraden C. Improving communication in the ICU using daily goals. Journal of Critical Care. 2003;**18**(2):71-75. DOI: 10.1053/jcrc.2003.50008

[21] Clinician-Patient Communication To Enhance Health Outcomes—Google Scholar [Internet]. Available from: https://scholar.google.com/scholar?hl=en&as_sdt=0%2C5&q=Clinician-Patient+Communication+To+Enhance+Health+Outcomes&btnG= [Accessed: June 1, 2018]

[22] Makoul G. Essential elements of communication in medical encounters: The Kalamazoo consensus statement. Academic Medicine. 2001;**76**(4):390-393. DOI: 10.1097/00001888-200104000-00021

[23] Levinson W, Hudak P, Tricco AC. A systematic review of surgeon–patient communication: Strengths and opportunities for improvement. Patient Education and Counseling. 2013;**93**(1):3-17. DOI: 10.1016/j.pec.2013.03.023

[24] Kaba R, Sooriakumaran P. The evolution of the doctor-patient relationship. International Journal of Surgery. 2007;**5**(1):57-65. DOI: 10.1016/j.ijsu.2006.01.005

[25] Maguire GP, Rutter DR. History-taking for medical students: I—Deficiencies in performance. The Lancet. 1976;**308**(7985):556-558. DOI: 10.1016/S0140-6736(76)91804-3

[26] Coulehan JL, Platt FW, Egener B, Frankel R, Lin C-T, Lown B, et al. "let me see if I have this right...": Words that help build empathy. Annals of Internal Medicine. 2001;**135**(3):221-227. DOI: 10.7326/0003-4819-135-3-200108070-00022

[27] Maguire P, Pitceathly C. Key communication skills and how to acquire them. BMJ. 2002;**325**(7366):697-700. DOI: 10.1136/bmj.325.7366.697

[28] Kalet AL, Janicik R, Schwartz M, Roses D, Hopkins MA, Riles T. Teaching communication skills on the surgery clerkship. Medical Education Online. 2005;**10**(1):4382. DOI: 10.3402/meo.v10i.4382

[29] Rudd RE. Health literacy skills of US adults. American Journal of Health Behavior. 2007;**31**(1):S8-S18. DOI: 10.5993/AJHB.31.s1.3

[30] Dreeben-Irimia O. Patient Education in Rehabilitation. Burlington, Massachusetts: Jones & Bartlett Publishers; 2010. ISBN 13: 9780763755447

[31] National Patient Safety Foundation [Internet]. Available from: http://www.ihi.org/resources/Pages/OtherWebsites/NationalPatientSafetyFoundation.aspx [Accessed: Jun 3, 2018]

[32] Barry MJ, Edgman-Levitan S. Shared decision making—The pinnacle of patient-centered care. The New England Journal of Medicine. 2012;**366**(9):780-781. DOI: 10.1056/NEJMp1109283

[33] Charles C, Gafni A, Whelan T. Shared decision-making in the medical encounter: What does it mean?(or it takes at least two to tango). Social Science & Medicine. 1997;**44**(5): 681-692. DOI: 10.1016/S0277-9536(96)00221-3

[34] Barry MJ, Edgman-Levitan S. Shared Decision Making — The Pinnacle of Patient-Centered Care. N Engl J Med. 2012 Feb 29;**366**(9):780-1

[35] Buckman R. Breaking bad news: Why is it still so difficult? British Medical Journal (Clinical Research Edition). 1984;**288**(6430):1597. DOI: 10.1136/bmj.288.6430.1597

[36] Baile WF, Buckman R, Lenzi R, Glober G, Beale EA, Kudelka AP. SPIKES—A six-step protocol for delivering bad news: Application to the patient with cancer. The Oncologist. 2000;**5**(4):302-311. DOI: 10.1634/theoncologist.5-4-302

[37] TeamStepps. Agency for Healthcare Research & Quality [Internet]. Available from: https://www.ahrq.gov/teamstepps/index.html [Accessed: June 3, 2018]

[38] Lencioni P. The Five Dysfunctions of a Team. A leadership Fable. California: Jossey Bass, San Francisco; 2002

[39] Haynes AB, Weiser TG, Berry WR, Lipsitz SR, Breizat A-HS, Dellinger EP, et al. A surgical safety checklist to reduce morbidity and mortality in a global population. The New England Journal of Medicine. 2009;**360**(5):491-499. DOI: 10.1056/NEJMsa0810119

[40] Van Klei WA, Hoff RG, Van Aarnhem E, Simmermacher RKJ, Regli LPE, Kappen TH, et al. Effects of the introduction of the WHO "surgical safety checklist" on in-hospital mortality: A cohort study. Annals of Surgery. 2012;**255**(1):44-49. DOI: 10.1097/SLA.0b013e31823779ae

[41] Weiser TG, Haynes AB, Lashoher A, Dziekan G, Boorman DJ, Berry WR, et al. Perspectives in quality: Designing the WHO surgical safety checklist. International Journal for Quality in Health Care. 2010;**22**(5):365-370. DOI: 10.1093/intqhc/mzq039

Chapter 4

Fundamentals of Medical Radiation Safety: Focus on Reducing Short-Term and Long-Term Harmful Exposures

Alex Alers, Philip Salen, Vikas Yellapu, Manish Garg, Charles Bendas, Nicholas Cardiges, Gregory Domer, Timothy Oskin, Jay Fisher and Stanislaw P. Stawicki

Additional information is available at the end of the chapter

http://dx.doi.org/10.5772/intechopen.85689

Abstract

This chapter provides an overview of key topics in the area of radiation safety. Three clinical vignettes will serve to frame the review of the literature around both diagnostic radiation exposure and the risk of radioisotope contamination. Advancement in medical technology is rarely innocuous, and the use of radiation as both means to diagnose and treat certain conditions is not an exception. It is very important for clinicians to review the basics of harmful medical radiation exposure since, although seldom encountered, treatment, and outcomes are time sensitive. The advent of newer technology and the widespread availability of equipment will only serve to increase the prevalence of potentially harmful medical radiation exposure. Moreover, this chapter aims to explore current multidisciplinary endeavors to provide safe and efficient use of radiation in medicine. Solely relying on the medical profession for development of safeguards against harmful medical radiation exposure would be an impossible task. This is why it is crucial for professionals such as health physicists, radiation safety enforcement officers, and policy-makers at the state, national, and international level to establish consensus guidelines aimed toward safe, reliable utilization of radiation in medicine. Part of this interdisciplinary approach needs to focus on accurate education of patients. A thorough assessment of acute radiation syndrome, including diagnosis, treatment, and prognostic indicators is also part of this chapter. Furthermore, principles of screening for, and protection from, radiation contamination are outlined. Finally, areas for further research are identified throughout the chapter. The discussion takes into account both US-based and International research and practice guidelines.

Keywords: diagnostic radiation exposure, patient safety, radiation exposure, radiation safety, radioisotope contamination, safety protocols

1. Introduction

Because of its low incidence, the risk of patient exposure to ionizing radiation is often underestimated—and underappreciated—as a patient safety (PS) threat across various healthcare settings. Consequently, the Joint Commission mandates that hospitals prepare for managing radiation-related risks in terms of protecting patients from unnecessary exposure, limiting any associated potential damage, monitoring the types and extent of radiation, and maintaining proficiency in decontamination procedures in cases of direct radioactive isotope contact [1, 2]. In terms of everyday healthcare facility functioning, there is a dual focus to ensure that radiation safety standards are met: (a) avoidance of unnecessary exposure including improper dosing and (b) assurance that radioactive material will be properly handled and disposed [2].

Regardless of the details or the mode of delivery, the intent of the treating team should always be the reduction in both short- and long-term radiation exposures [3]. It has been recommended by different organizations and authors that radiation exposure reduction (RER) efforts encompass both pre-procedural and procedural phases of treatment [4, 5]. The use of radiation for diagnostic or therapeutic indications (RDTI) has clear benefits when appropriately directed and supervised. However, serious errors, prolonged or repeated exposures, and lack of supervision can be associated with significant adverse consequences, including the risk of acute radiation sickness, malignancy, and death [6–10]. **Table 1** [top section] lists the

Side effect	Frequency	Minimum exposure amount (Rads)
Hyperpigmentation/erythema	>50%	50–200
Mild fatigue	>50%	50–200
Mild myelosuppression	>50%	50–200
Skin desquamation	<10%	100
Mild nausea/vomiting/diarrhea	<10%	100–400
Intractable vomiting/diarrhea	90%	>400
Comparison of alternative units of measure		**Conversion factor**
1 Rad		0.01 Joule/kg; 0.01 Gray; 0.01 Sv
1 Millirad		0.00001 Joule/kg; 0.00001 Gray; 0.00001 Sv
1 Milligray; 1 Centigray; 1 Decigray; 1 Dekagray		0.1; 1; 10; 1000 Rads, etc. (respectively)
1 Coulomb/kg		3876 Roentgen; 3875 Parker; 3875 Rep
1 Millicoulomb/kg		3.876 Roentgen*
1 Microcoulomb/kg		0.003876 Roentgen*
1 Tissue Roentgen		1 Roentgen

kg = kilogram; Sv = Sievert; * = same applies for Parker and Rep units.

Table 1. Approximate incidence of adverse effect at different radiation exposures measured in Rads.

approximate incidence of adverse effects at various levels of radiation exposure (measured in Rads). In addition, comparative descriptions of alternative radiation units of measure are provided for the reader in the lower section of **Table 1**. The latter measure is intended to reduce the confusion often encountered due to multiple naming conventions in this area of science.

An important distinction must be made between radiation exposure and radioactive contamination. Radiation exposure refers to a person receiving energy in the form of waves or particles from an external source or from internal contamination [9, 10]. To prevent harm to the patient, the duration of exposure is carefully controlled. To prevent harm to the radiology technician, distance and shielding from source are employed [11, 12]. In contrast, a contaminated person has radioactive material on (or inside) the body secondary to ingestion, inhalation or deposition on the body surface. Thus, contamination can be classified as internal or external. Most patients exposed to radiation are not contaminated [13]. Radiation can be measured in SI unit Gray (Gy), which represents the absorption of one joule of radiation energy per kilogram of matter. In order to reflect the degree of radioactive contamination in human tissue, the unit of Sievert (Sv) us usually employed. The following clinical vignettes will illustrate both radiation exposure (#1) and contamination (#2 and #3). For the purposes of our chapter, the reader should be familiar with the three general types of radiation, including the associated energetic characteristics and shielding capacity (**Table 2**). In addition, various levels of radiation exposure (measured in millisieverts) including the typical associated contextual settings are shown in **Figure 1**.

1.1. Clinical vignette #1

Over a period of months, numerous patients who underwent computed tomography (CT) perfusion scans of the brain at different hospitals across a wide geographic area reported vague complaints of oddly shaped patterns of unexpected hair loss. Reportedly, the mostly band-like areas of alopecia appeared within 1–2 weeks following each patient's CT study. Some patients began complaining of new onset memory loss and/or difficulty keeping balance while walking. Given the unusual pattern of clinical signs and symptoms, as well as the isolated nature of occurrences, it took months before the connection was made between CT perfusion scans and what turned out to be significant radiation overdoses. When the true scope of the problem became evident, hundreds of patients were identified as having received approximately eight times the expected levels of radiation. It appeared that the root cause for the above occurrences may be faulty programming of CT scanner devices. A nationwide statement of caution was issued by the FDA, urging hospitals across the US to

Type of radiation	Penetrating energy	Penetrating capacity in human body	Shielding capacity
Alpha (α)	Low	Epidermis	Dissipates in air
Beta (β)	Intermediate	Soft tissue	Sheet of paper
Gamma (γ)	High	Bones and organs	Lead

Table 2. Types of ionizing radiation, with corresponding levels of penetration and preferred shielding characteristics.

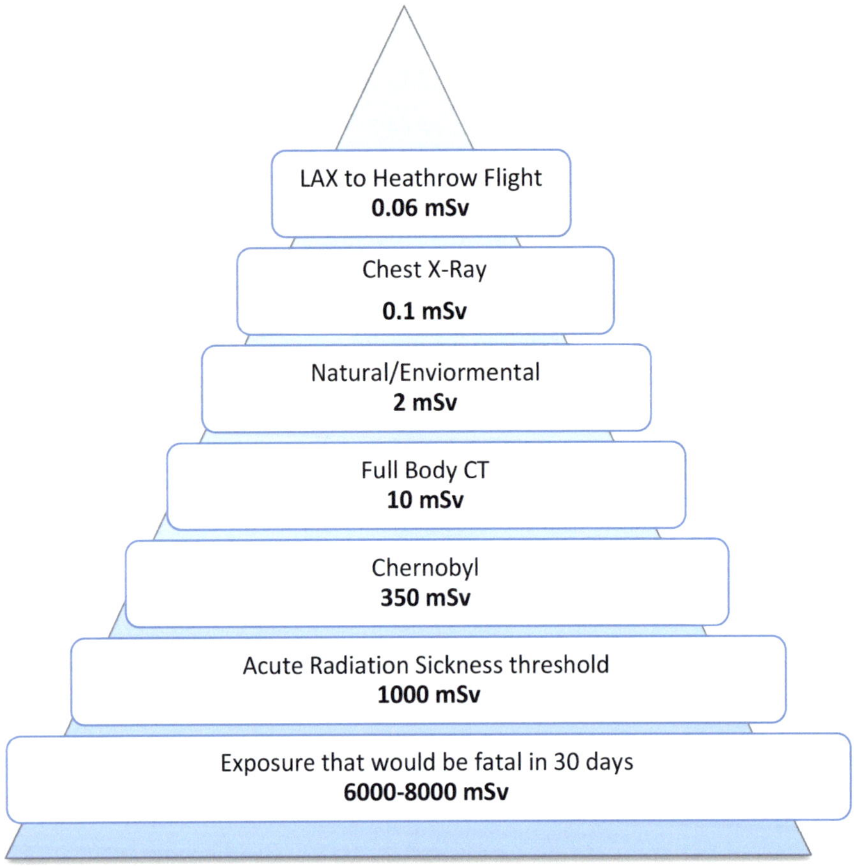

Figure 1. Different levels of radiation exposure, measured in millisieverts (mSv) and the associated biological manifestations.

review institutional CT scan logs to check radiation dosage levels and data regarding applicable adherence to established dosing protocols [14, 15]. In response to the above events, the first state law in the US aimed at protecting patients from excessive radiation exposure during CT scans was signed into law by Gov. Arnold Schwarzenegger of California [16]. In addition to providing an accreditation mandate for CT scanners, the bill also requires that radiation dose be recorded on the scanned image in a patient's medical record, and that radiation overdoses be reported to patients, treating physicians, and the state Department of Public Health [16].

1.2. Clinical vignette #2

In 1987, improperly abandoned hospital radiation equipment in Goiania, Brazil, led to the contamination of a large number of people. During the post-incident review, it was discovered that an unused irradiation machine was left behind when a privately owned healthcare facility moved. The device was subsequently stolen by a group of young men who sold it to a scrap metal dealer. During the disassembly of the medical equipment, a broken capsule of the highly radioactive cesium-137 was accidentally smashed, along with its lead enclosure, liberating "shiny bluish dust which glowed in the dark" [17]. Unaware of the danger, numerous individuals associated with the scrap metal yard owner came into contact with the radioactive powder. The most seriously affected victims developed alopecia, cutaneous burns, vomiting and diarrhea. The governmental response was slow at first, due mainly to the lack of recognition of the magnitude and the urgency of the situation. Experts from the Soviet Union and the US were involved in the subsequent management and containment of the radioactive risk. The incident was thought to be the most serious of its kind at the time, with 240 documented cases of contamination, 20 hospitalizations, and 4 fatalities [17, 18].

1.3. Clinical vignette #3

In 1992, an unexpected discovery of radioactive waste was made by a regional disposal company in Indiana, Pennsylvania [9, 19]. Subsequent investigation by the US National Regulatory Commission (NRC) found that in November of 1992, a local clinic in Indiana, Pennsylvania treated a patient with high-dose brachytherapy using an iridium-192 radioactive source [20]. It was determined that the treatment was not completed due to equipment-related issues. Unknown to the operators, the source wire became fractured and remained in the patient. Investigators discovered that the required radiation survey at the end of the treatment was not performed. The patient was discharged to a nursing home and died 5 days later. Unaware of the danger, nursing home staff removed the source-containing catheter and disposed of it as biohazardous waste [9]. The source was identified during routine radiation surveillance by the waste disposal company. In addition to being a contributor to the index patient's death, more than 90 individuals may have been exposed to the radioactive material, with doses ranging from <0.05 to >2.55 rem [20].

2. The magnitude of the "silent" problem

Difficult to identify at the time of the initial exposure, radiation injury tends to present in a delayed fashion. Radiation injury also tends to be low on a typical differential diagnosis list as most cases tend to involve unintentional (and unrecognized) exposure. As demonstrated by our three vignettes, the uncommon occurrence of harmful medical radiation exposure (HMRE) can originate as a result of various types of PS error; both of omission and of commission [21]. In addition, radiation-related PS issues can result from lack of adequate oversight at both institutional level (e.g., absent safety procedures) and governmental level (e.g., lack of applicable laws, regulations, or enforcement) [9, 22, 23].

Complexities associated with HMRE prompted an important discussion regarding the nature and the content of the informed consent process, specifically as it relates to medical radiation exposure [24]. The true gravity of such considerations is exemplified by the known association between cumulative radiation exposure and the incremental risk of malignancy following repeated CT imaging episodes [25]. Moreover, compared to the adult population, the overall risk is significantly greater for pediatric patients [26].

3. Biological manifestations of HMRE

Two broad categories of clinical (e.g., biologic) effects of radiation, specific to the contexts of radiation therapy or accidental isotope exposure, include deterministic injuries and stochastic injuries. Deterministic injuries manifest as radiation-induced escalation of normal physiologic apoptosis resulting in increased death of essential cells with resultant tissue and organ dysfunction [27]. These types of injuries occur when large numbers of cells become damaged and, as a result, die immediately or shortly after irradiation [28]. Dermatoligic post-exposure injury can range from "local erythema" to "skin necrosis" [28]. Estimation of dosage is measured in the units of Gy, with 0–2 Gy associated with no biological effects; 2–5 Gy causing transient erythema (<2 weeks), followed by epilation (2–8 weeks) and recovery (6–52 weeks); 5–10 Gy associated with prolonged erythema (up to 8 weeks), epilation (2–8 weeks), and recovery (6–52 weeks); 10–15 Gy exposure causes transient erythema (<2 weeks), dry/moist desquamation (2–8 weeks), followed by permanent epilation (6–52 weeks) and finally atrophy (>40 weeks); and >15 Gy being associated with acute ulceration (<2 weeks), moist desquamation (2–8 weeks), dermal necrosis (6–52 weeks), and eventual surgery (>40 weeks) [28]. **Table 3** outlines the above exposure levels in a systematized fashion.

Stochastic effects manifest as cellular carcinogenesis and result from radiation induced mutations in genetic material of cells including germ cells [27]. For stochastic injuries, post-radiation damage becomes the key determinant of clinically apparent, usually long-term manifestation [28]. Such effects also depend on the type/activity of the isotope involved. More specifically, these kinds of injuries have a linear nonthreshold dose that may lead to radiation-induced malignancy and/or heritable genetic defects [28]. Estimation of dosage from radiologic studies utilizes the units of Sieverts (Sv), with procedures such as dual-isotope SPECT (24 mSv) and CT angiography (19 mSv), carrying the highest effective radiation doses [28]. Of note, victims of the Chernobyl disaster were exposed to a maximum radioactivity of 300–450 mSv/h within a 15 km radius. The individuals that had suffered from radiation are suspected to have received a minimum of 0.8–2 Gy (80–200 Rad) dose [28].

Radiation dose (Gy)	Possible adverse reaction	Timeline
0–2	No effect	
2–5	Transient erythema	<2 weeks
5–10	Prolonged erythema	<8 weeks
10–15	Dry/moist desquamation leading to permanent epilation	2–8 weeks → 6–52 weeks
>15	Acute ulceration leading to desquamation and dermal necrosis	<2 weeks → 6–52 weeks

Table 3. Post-exposure deterministic injury shown with radiation dose in Gray units and the typical timeline associated with the appearance of adverse effects.

4. Regulatory mechanisms and safety enforcement

The first line of ensuring safety is the presence of organizational policies and procedures pertaining to HMRE as well as the handling of radioisotope-containing medical materials, both at the departmental and institutional levels [29–31]. In addition to applicable policies and procedures that are harmonized to prevailing laws and regulations, organizations also employ radiation safety experts in the role of Radiation Safety Officer (or functional equivalent thereof) to ensure the maintenance of appropriate legal and procedural compliance [31–33]. Any HMRE events that are deemed reportable to appropriate local, regional, or national authorities are handled by the Radiation Safety Officer. In addition, employees who work around radiation equipment and/or interact with medical radioisotopes must wear radiation monitoring badges that help quantify levels of healthcare worker exposure [34, 35]. Some general considerations of how appropriate policies and procedures can help protect the well-being of both patients and healthcare workers include [7, 32, 36–38]:

- In diagnostic radiography, the use of hardwired "safety prompts" helps facilitate double-checking of the expected radiation dosage; also, it is important to ensure the presence of appropriate warning lights, such as "X-ray in progress" and sufficiently labeled facilities with caution signs
- Ensuring that the delivery process of therapeutic radiation is appropriately structured, including thorough planning, simulated application, and the presence of built-in cross-checks (e.g., two or more experts sign-off on the final therapeutic plan, including the physician, the physicist, and a dosimetrist)
- Monitoring of cumulative monthly radiation exposure and limiting further exposure for those employees who exceeded established thresholds
- Protocolized monitoring of medical waste for the presence of radioactivity, both at the site of origin (e.g., the hospital) and at the destination (e.g., landfill)

In the European Union and associated countries, the Euratom Treaty recommends that a patient examination and clinical justification are provided before a referral is made to a radiologist or a nuclear medicine expert. Moreover, nonionizing radiation is preferred whenever it will provide comparable information to that obtained by means of ionizing radiation [39]. For example, an ultrasound or magnetic resonance imaging (MRI) may provide the same desired information as a CT, without the need for ionizing radiation [40]. Additional safety enforcement strategies include: safety checklists to verify the patient and study being performed; radiation dose customization utilizing the patient's weight, age, medical history, and intended body segment to be scanned/imaged; and decision support systems which provide ordering physicians an opportunity to answer questions regarding their patients and consider alternatives to ionizing diagnostics [40].

The US Food and Drug Administration (FDA) has partnered with other organizations to promote education and communication regarding radiation safety to patients and medical professionals

[41]. Among their resources, the FDA collaborated with the National Council on Radiation Protection and Measurement to communicate the risk of radiation exposure with patients, particularly imaging involving young children [41, 42]. The FDA advocates for patient and healthcare provider awareness via the Image Wisely and Image Gently radiation risk campaigns, as well as with the International Atomic Energy Agency's "Radiation Protection of Patients" website [41, 43, 44]. The FDA has also advocated for patient and healthcare provider tools to reduce radiation exposure. One particular innovative safety tool is the "Patient Medical Imaging Record Card", which was developed by the FDA in collaboration with Image Wisely [41, 43]. The card can be used to track patient imaging studies by date, type, and location to prevent unnecessary repeat ionizing radiation exposures [41]. Looking toward the future, this card would ideally be integrated into the patient's electronic health record and stored in a nationally accessible database for healthcare providers, such as the Federal Data service Hub, which is established by the Affordable Care Act and backed by the Health and Human Services department [45].

The US Nuclear Regulatory Commission was established with The Energy Reorganization Act of 1974 to license and regulate the civilian use of radioactive materials to protect public health and safety and the environment. It is in charge of overseeing nuclear reactors, security, and materials as well as radioactive waste. The commission sets rules and licensing, enforces those rules, evaluates facilities, and provides support and logistics for incident response. Some aspects of management and regulation of certain radioactive materials have been granted to Agreement States [46].

5. Radiation injury

Although most individuals exposed to radiation contamination are not symptomatic, the consequences of such exposures tend to result in long-term sequelae [47–50]. Providers should be aware of signs and symptoms of radiation injury so that such occurrences can be readily recognized, contained, and victims treated promptly [51, 52]. As demonstrated in our *Clinical Vignette #1*, acute HMRE tends to have organ-specific, regional anatomic manifestations (e.g., pneumonitis, lung fibrosis, gastric ulceration, and radiation proctitis) [52–54]. Systemic manifestations (e.g., acute radiation syndrome) are extremely rare in the healthcare setting and usually involve direct exposures of patients, workers, or otherwise unsuspecting individuals, to the radioactive isotope material, as outlined in our *clinical vignette #2* [18, 55] and *clinical vignette #3* [9, 19, 20].

Acute radiation syndrome (ARaS), unlike radiation injury, is a systemic entity that occurs very rarely in the healthcare setting. It usually involves some form of equipment failure, radioactive isotope release, criminal activity/theft, or inappropriate disposal of equipment or isotope(s) [9, 18–20, 55]. Because ARaS may be the only overt "manifestation" of a major radioactive breach, it is critical that it is promptly recognized, and that it leads to a thorough investigation into associated events. Symptoms of ARaS evolve over time in distinct phases. The duration of each phase and the time of its onset will be approximately inversely proportional to the dose [56]. An initial prodromal phase, with symptoms such as nausea, vomiting, weakness, and fatigue, typically develops within hours to days after exposure of the

Syndrome	Hematopoietic	Gastrointestinal	Cardiovascular/neurovascular
Dose	>0.3–0.7 Gy	>6–10 Gy	>20–50 Gy
Prodromal stage (minutes—2 days)	Anorexia, nausea/vomiting	Anorexia, severe nausea, vomiting, cramps, and diarrhea	Extreme nervousness and confusion, severe nausea, vomiting, watery diarrhea, loss of consciousness and burning sensation of the skin
Latent stage	Patient appears well for 1–6 weeks	Patient appears and feels well for less than a week	Patient may return to partial functionality (often lasts less than several hours)
Manifest illness stage	Anorexia, fever, and malaise Drop in all blood cell counts Primary cause of death is infection and hemorrhage Most deaths within a few months Survival rate is inversely proportional to dose	Malaise, anorexia, severe diarrhea, fever, dehydration, and electrolyte imbalance Death occurs within 2 weeks after exposure	Watery diarrhea, convulsions, and coma Onset occurs 5–6 hours after exposure Death occurs within 3 days of exposure
Recovery	Full recovery for large percentage of patients from a few weeks to 2 years after exposure Death may occur in some individuals at 1.2 Gy The $LD_{50/60}$ is 2.5 to 5 Gy	The LD_{100} is about 10 Gy	No recovery expected

Table 4. Acute radiation syndrome: most common manifestations [13].

whole body to radiation exceeding 0.7 Gray (Gy). ARaS manifests most acutely and severely in the hematopoietic, gastrointestinal, and cardiovascular/neurovascular systems [27, 57]. Radiation-induced gastrointestinal manifestations of ARaS manifest as nausea, vomiting, and bloody diarrhea. Severe dermatological injury with burns, desquamation, epilation, and ulceration can occur after significant radiation exposure even in the absence of ARaS [58], as exemplified by our *clinical vignette #1*. The above manifestations are summarized in **Table 4**.

6. Protection from and screening for radiation contamination

The general principles of protection from radiation injury depend upon four factors: distance, time, shielding, and removal or containment of contamination [27]. When caring for potential radiation contaminated patients, healthcare personnel must minimize the duration of exposure to a source, maximize the distance from source, and establish effective shielding from the source. Identification of the presence of radioactive contamination on or within a patient mandates early removal/containment in order to forestall further damage and contamination [27]. In cases similar to the Goiania incident, hand-held Geiger counters must be utilized in order to focus on accurately identifying anatomic areas of contamination unique to each individual [1]. Substantial exposure of emergency responders and clinicians caring for potentially heavily contaminated patients may occur. Emergency medical services and clinicians must use caution and adhere to strict precautions for managing hazardous materials to prevent inadvertent contamination of themselves and others [27]. Personnel should wear radiation dosimeters, sealed in clear, airtight plastic bags, and worn outside the clothing to allow rapid assessment and early detection of contamination. Workers and work areas should undergo repeated surveillance with radiation detectors at appropriate intervals [1, 27].

7. Laboratory evaluation of acute radiation injury

In cases of more significant exposure, ARaS manifests initially through the hematopoietic system as blood marrow tissues are highly radiosensitive [27]. Of all the components of hematopoiesis, circulating lymphocytes have the most radiosensitive cell lines and provides a useful laboratory tool to screen for the severity of the radiation sickness early in observation (**Figure 2**) [56]. After whole body exposure above 0.5 Gy, the rapid fall in lymphocyte number starts within hours, and the lymphocyte depletion is proportional to the dose between 1 and 10 Gy [56]. GM-CSF may be helpful for the recovery of the bone marrow function after clinically significant radiation exposure [57]. Lymphocyte depletion kinetics serves as the single best estimator of radiation exposure and clinical outcome [27]. A decrease in absolute lymphocyte levels may be observed at whole-body doses as low as 100 mSv, but clinically significant response may not be seen below 1–2 Sv. Depending on the absorbed dose, such changes can begin within hours of exposure, so it is recommended that an immediate complete blood count with differential is performed as a baseline and then every 6–12 hours thereafter for 2–3 days [27]. An elevated serum amylase provides a supplementary piece of information that may also be an early sign of serious radiation exposure involving the head and neck. The results of this test are nonspecific; however, and they may also reflect alcohol intake, a stress response, trauma

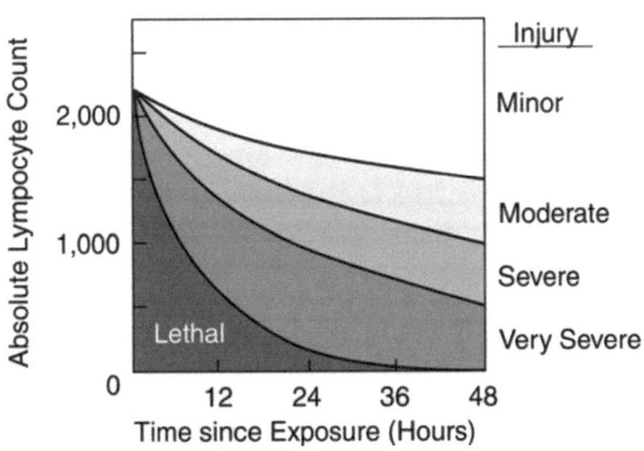

Figure 2. Time-dependent lymphocyte depletion kinetics following either severe or moderate radiation exposures. As early as 6–12 hours following exposure, there may be some indication of the severity of the exposure [35].

http://dx.doi.org/10.5772/intechopen.85689

to the face or abdomen, or other factors [27]. In addition, the presence of nausea and vomiting within several (usually around 4) hours of exposure may also be diagnostically helpful.

8. Measuring severity of radiation dose

Similar to other toxicological phenomena, determining the potential harm of radiation exposure mandates consideration of three factors: dose of radiation exposure, tissue or surface area exposed, and duration of exposure. Whole body radiation exposure to 4 or 5 Sv (or Gy) imparts potentially lethal effects, while an extremity can tolerate several times that exposure [27]. General measures of radiation exposure (e.g., fluoroscopy time) have low utility and accuracy [28]. At this juncture, it is important to introduce the concept of KERMA, or "Kinetic Energy Released in Matter", which is a measure of energy delivered (or dose) [28]. Air-KERMA is the KERMA measured in air (e.g., low scatter environment) [28]. More useful methods of determining radiation administered include: (a) total air-KERMA (exposure) at pre-specified reference point, (b) air-KERMA area product, and (c) peak skin dose or the maximum dose received by any local area of patient skin [28, 59]. See **Figures 3–5** for further information.

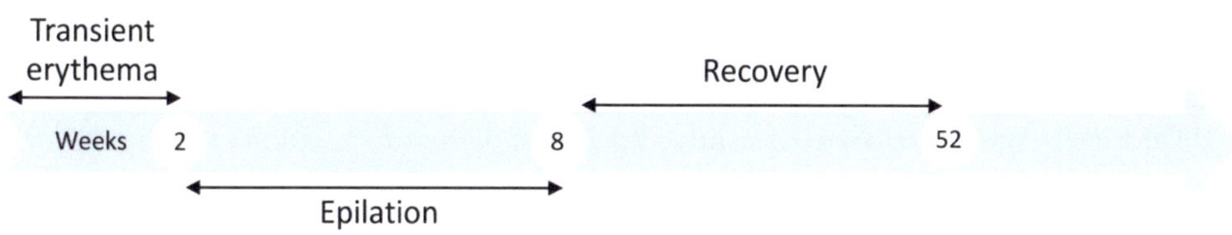

Figure 3. Timeline for post exposure injury for dosage of 2–5 Gy.

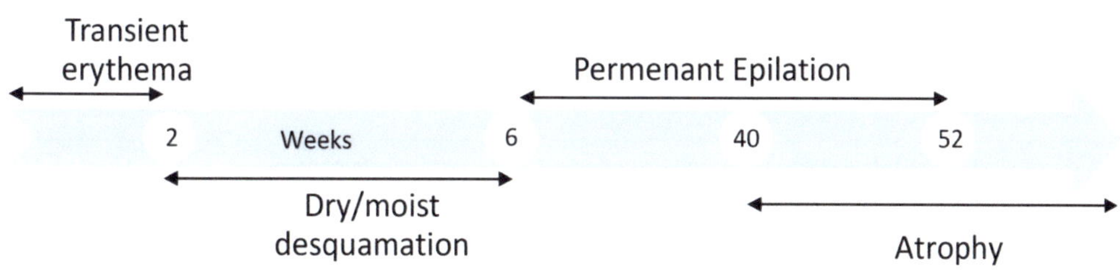

Figure 4. Timeline for post exposure injury for dosage of 10–15 Gy.

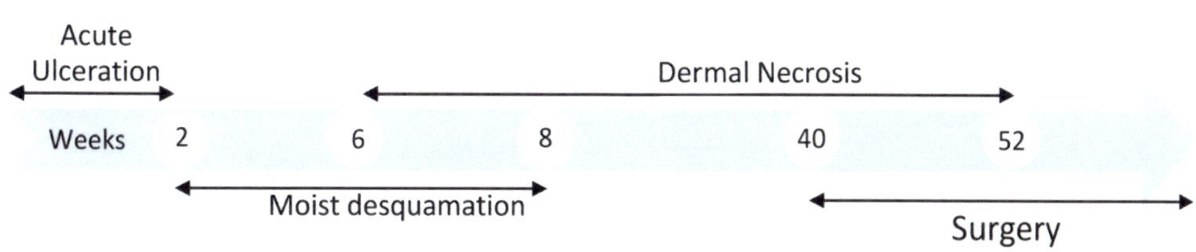

Figure 5. Timeline for post exposure injury for dosage >15 Gy.

9. Patient exposure to radiation

A point of concern among care providers and parents is the risk of radiation exposure from medical imaging, especially in the pediatric population. Epidemiologic studies have shown that *in utero* exposure to radiation is associated with higher incidence of pediatric cancers, but data related to rates of pediatric and adult cancers are relatively scarce [60]. In recent years, CT scanning has become the favored imaging modality in many clinical scenarios and is likely to see even further increases in use going forward [61–63]. As such, CT utilization in pediatrics has increased markedly over the last 20 years. Over 85 million CT scans are performed annually in the United States, with 5–11% of these performed on children [64]. Before we embark on further discussion, important dose-related information in the context of diagnostic testing is provided in **Table 5**.

A typical CT scan of the head of a child carries an average dose of 2–2.5 millisieverts (mSv) of radiation. CT imaging of the chest and abdomen carries doses averaging 3–4 and 5–6 mSv, respectively. The actual dose administered differs from the more nebulous effective dose, as other factors make the amount of radiation exposure more meaningful in children than adults. The effective radiation doses received by children are about 50% higher than those received by adults for similar imaging studies due to smaller body sizes and radiation attenuation [66, 67]. Up to an age of 10, children are approximately three times more sensitive to radiation than adults, which is why longer life expectancy coupled with organ systems that are still developing disproportionately increases the relative burden of pediatric radiation exposure [67–69].

Several studies have attempted to answer questions regarding specific childhood cancer risks associated with radiation exposure. Two studies showed increased incidence of pediatric leukemia in children with medical radiation exposure; however, these studies used retrospective questionnaire data and their result as inconsistent with older data [70, 71]. Certain genetic phenotypes might make some children more sensitive to the effects of radiation and risk of acute lymphocytic leukemia [72]. Very limited data exist on CT-attributable risk of

Relative radiation level	**Adult effective dose estimate range (mSv)**	**Pediatric effective dose estimate range (mSv)**	**Example examinations**
O	0	0	Ultrasound; MRI
☢	<0.1	<0.03	Chest X-ray; hand X-rays
☢☢	0.1–1	0.03–0.3	Pelvis X-ray; mammography
☢☢☢	1–10	0.3–3	Abdomen CT; nuclear medicine bone scan
☢☢☢☢	10–30	3–10	Abdomen CT with and without contrast; whole body PET
☢☢☢☢☢	30–100	10–30	CTA chest abdomen pelvis with contrast; transjugular intrahepatic portosystemic shunt placement

Table 5. Relative radiation level designations along with associated effective adult and pediatric doses, as well as imaging examinations that correspond to said levels [65].

solid tumors in children. There is weak evidence regarding the association between radiation exposure and such occurrences (e.g., pediatric astrocytoma and Ewing's sarcoma), but this connection is in no way definitive [60].

Data regarding the lifetime risk of cancers appear to be more robust. A large retrospective cohort study reviewed >175,000 patients from the NHS registry in England [26]. The authors noted a positive association between dose of radiation from CT imaging and leukemia and brain tumors. They found relative risk of leukemia to be 3.18 in patients who received more than 30 mSv of cumulative radiation. Similarly, they found an increased relative risk of brain cancer to be 2.82 in pediatric patients who received cumulative dosing of 50 mSv or more [26]. The caveat to these data, however, is that these are rare cancers to begin with, thus the absolute relative risk increase is very small. Although the relative risk of brain cancer may nearly triple with significant cumulative radiation exposure, the absolute risk is still exceedingly small. Based on robust statistical models, for every 100,000 skull/brain CT scans in 5-year-old children, eight brain/central nervous system cancers and four cases of leukemia would result [73]. The same study estimates that 100,000 chest CT scans would lead to an excess of 31 thyroid cancers, 55 breast malignancies, and 1 leukemia case [73]. Consequently, the lifetime risk of cancers, although small, should be discussed with parents of children undergoing CT scanning. Although these studies are largely safe in children, unnecessary exposure to radiation should still be avoided, and diagnostic tests not utilizing ionizing radiation should be used whenever possible. The medical necessity of imaging should be weighed against the relatively small risk of harm when determining the appropriateness of these studies. Again, the greatest risk of cancer appears to exist when children are exposed to cumulative doses of radiation greater than 30–50 mSv.

10. Pregnancy and reproductive health considerations

According to the American College of Radiology, no single diagnostic X-ray study or procedure results in radiation exposure sufficient to threaten the well-being of the pregnant patient, the developing embryo, or the fetus [74]. In fact, diagnostic radiation exposures during pregnancy may be safer than the frequent concerns over *in utero* radiation exposure suggest [75]. Moreover, the utilization of diagnostic radiological imaging may entail more benefit than risk in the evaluation of certain maternal injuries or illnesses [76]. As much attention should focus on limiting diagnostic radiation exposure of the gravid woman's breast tissue, to prevent carcinogenesis, as on limiting radiation exposure of the fetus [77, 78]. In the setting of pregnancy, radiation exposure should be limited to 1 mGy during the first trimester, with teratogenicity risk being elevated at 5 mGy [79]. In addition, iodine-containing contrast media may lead to hypothyroidism in the fetus, an additional consideration when performing radiographic studies utilizing contrast material [79]. Counseling of the patient by the referring clinician and by the radiologist is essential in providing informed consent as the benefits and risks of procedures can be opaque and the decision may impart lasting consequences [80]. Impacting 5–7% of all pregnancies, trauma represents an important cause of nonobstetric maternal morbidity and mortality [81]. Consequently, the risk-benefit equation regarding diagnostic imaging in this particular setting is somewhat different, with the mantra that the best way to ensure fetal wellbeing is to aggressively treat the mother [82].

11. Radiation exposure as low as reasonably achievable (ALARA)

Literature suggesting that accrual of cumulative radiation exposures from diagnostic radiological studies, such as CT scans or fluoroscopy, over the course of patients' lifetimes puts them at risk for the potential carcinogenic risks of radiation [83, 84]. One example here comes from the area of endovascular interventional procedures. Since the introduction of endovascular therapy in the late 1980s, there has been incredible growth in this group of procedural modalities. In fact, endovascular procedures have increased approximately 400% over the past decade [85]. The applicability and medical advancements of this form of therapy have revolutionized treatment of our patients. However, there has been an associated cost, including substantial risk of ionizing radiation exposure [86]. Some of the pioneers of endovascular therapy have succumbed to the deleterious consequence of ionizing radiation [87]. Radiation safety practices have made tremendous advances since the discovery of Roentgen's X-rays over 120 years ago. Early practitioners were focused on patient outcomes and providing minimally invasive methods to treat complex disease processes. These sacrifices of early practitioners led to our awareness and knowledge that now allows us to perform truly remarkable treatments to benefit our patients. A number of very practical steps can be taken to reduce radiation exposure to patients, operators, and staff [88, 89]. Awareness itself can be an effective first step in reducing exposure. Once awareness of the problem exists, we can then work to educate and enact training and methodology to achieve maximal safety to our patients and ourselves. However, despite the available data, there remains a significant safety deficit. In 2014, a survey of US vascular surgery trainees found 45% had no formal radiation safety training, 74% were unaware of the radiation safety policy for pregnant females, 48% did not know their radiation safety officer's contact information, and 43% were unaware of the acceptable yearly levels of radiation exposure [90]. However, an important observation was that the trainees who felt their attendings were applying ALARA techniques were much more likely to do so themselves. Therefore, it is incumbent on those of us providing training to the next generation of caregivers to set an example of excellence and expect the same from our trainees. Only by expecting excellence can we hope to achieve superior safety for our patients and ourselves.

Advocates for radiation safety recommend exposing patients, especially children, to as little radiation as possible. This is embodied within the concept of "as low as reasonably achievable" (ALARA) in the context of radiation exposure [84]. As such, ALARA addresses the role for healthcare providers, particularly those caring for children, in reducing exposure to radiation while maintaining the reliability of the diagnostic radiology modality [91]. Multiple methods can be used to achieve ALARA including: adjusting the amount of radiation in the diagnostic study based on patient weight, considering alternative modalities such as sonography or magnetic resonance imaging, enhancing shielding with thyroid or breast shields, focusing on the suspicious area with focused or limited view diagnostic imaging, and discouraging repeat CT scan studies [91]. In one example, although noninvasive multi-slice cardiac-computed tomography angiography (CCTA) can accurately screen for coronary ischemia, its widespread utilization has generated concern because of potential diagnostic radiation exposure. Utilization of a radiation dose reduction program in concert with limiting the image acquisition window for CCTA has demonstrated marked reduction, more than 50%, in estimated radiation doses in a statewide registry without impairment of image quality [83]. In another example, appendicitis represents the most common disease process resulting in increased CT scan utilization in children over the last two decades. Clinical practice guidelines advocating for "abdominal sonography first" for the evaluation of appendicitis have demonstrated comparable diagnostic accuracy to CT scan imaging, while reducing CT scan utilization and thus radiation exposure [91]. The Pediatric Emergency Care Applied Research Network collaborative development of a clinical decision guideline for pediatric head trauma is another example of research helping to reduce the medical radiation footprint by reliably identifying patients at low risk for clinically important traumatic brain injuries, for whom CT can routinely be obviated [92].

12. Safety protocols

Careful adherence to existing PS protocols, including active surveillance for any signs and/or symptoms of HMRE, is among the most important considerations for facilities/departments providing diagnostic and/or therapeutic radiation services [28]. In addition to direct radiation, the formation of X-ray image is inherently associated with some degree of "scattered radiation" that is the principal source of exposure to the patient and medical staff [28]. This "scatter" increases with both intensity of the X-ray beam and the size of the exposed field [28]. Any hospital employing medical radiation needs to have an infrastructure to support protocols for every step of the way throughout the application of said radiation including patient and healthcare worker safety, proper identification and dosing, and waste management of materials in order to prevent contamination.

13. Conclusions

The power to harness ionizing radiation for medical uses has a history spanning more than a century. Although its positive impact on the modern-day prowess of the diagnostician is unquestionable, great care must be taken in order to not abuse this technology. Diagnostic imaging with ionizing radiation seems poised to be part of the medical armamentarium for the foreseeable future. Further research is required in all aspects of this field, including more efficient protocols for delivery, custom-tailoring therapy which takes into account the patients' makeup, potential short-term and long-term harmful effects, the prediction and prevention of harm and better safeguards for dosimetry not only for patients but also for healthcare workers. Greater strides must be achieved in the realm of oversight and standardization of practice, as well as a comprehensive, nonpunitive reporting system for adverse events. A multidisciplinary approach from health physicists, radiation safety personnel, and clinicians is paramount for the management of contamination events and for the safe and accurate use of both diagnostic and therapeutic medical radiation. The key for this technology going forward is for education to be widespread among all levels of healthcare, from patients and their families to healthcare providers and policy makers. Research and public health information dissemination will go hand-in-hand throughout the next century of medical radiation use.

Author details

Alex Alers[1], Philip Salen[2], Vikas Yellapu[6], Manish Garg[3], Charles Bendas[1], Nicholas Cardiges[4], Gregory Domer[5], Timothy Oskin[5], Jay Fisher[5] and Stanislaw P. Stawicki[6]*

*Address all correspondence to: stawicki.ace@gmail.com

1 Department of Surgery, St. Luke's Level I Regional Trauma Center, St. Luke's University Health Network, Bethlehem, Pennsylvania, USA

2 Department of Emergency Medicine, St. Luke's University Health Network, Bethlehem, Pennsylvania, USA

3 Department of Emergency Medicine, Temple University School of Medicine, Philadelphia, Pennsylvania, USA

4 Department of Radiation Oncology, St. Luke's University Health Network, Bethlehem, Pennsylvania, USA

5 Heart and Vascular Center, Division of Vascular Surgery, St. Luke's University Health Network, Bethlehem, Pennsylvania, USA

6 Department of Research and Innovation, St. Luke's University Health Network, Bethlehem, Pennsylvania, USA

References

[1] Salen P et al. A randomized, double-blind, sham-controlled trial comparing two screening devices for radiation contamination. Academic Emergency Medicine. 2010;**17**(9): 1020-1023

[2] Almén A, Valentin J. 5.3 applied radiological protection. In: Fundamentals and Data in Radiobiology, Radiation Biophysics, Dosimetry and Medical Radiological Protection. Berlin Heidelberg: Springer-Verlag; 2012. pp. 261-287

[3] Douglas PS et al. Developing an action plan for patient radiation safety in adult cardiovascular medicine. Circulation. Cardiovascular Imaging. 2012;**5**(3):400-414

[4] Amis ES et al. American College of Radiology white paper on radiation dose in medicine. Journal of the American College of Radiology. 2007;**4**(5):272-284

[5] Dauer LT et al. Fears, feelings, and facts: Interactively communicating benefits and risks of medical radiation with patients. American Journal of Roentgenology. 2011;**196**(4):756-761

[6] Hendee WR, O'Connor MK. Radiation risks of medical imaging: Separating fact from fantasy. Radiology. 2012;**264**(2):312-321

[7] Bogdanich W. Radiation Offers New Cures, and Ways to Do Harm. New York: The New York Times; 2010. p. 23

[8] Leuraud K et al. Ionising radiation and risk of death from leukaemia and lymphoma in radiation-monitored workers (INWORKS): An international cohort study. The Lancet Haematology. 2015;**2**(7):e276-e281

[9] Dicus CGJ. Materials Safety and Regulation; 1997

[10] Hendee WR. Real and perceived risks of medical radiation exposure. Western Journal of Medicine. 1983;**138**(3):380

[11] JCS Joint Working Group. Guidelines for radiation safety in interventional cardiology (JCS 2006). Circulation Journal. 2010;**74**(12):2760-2785

[12] Thompson MA. Maintaining a proper perspective of risk associated with radiation exposure. Journal of Nuclear Medicine Technology. 2001;**29**(3):137-142

[13] CDC. Acute Radiation Syndrome: A Fact Sheet for Clinicians. 2018. Available from: https://emergency.cdc.gov/radiation/arsphysicianfactsheet.asp [Accessed: December 15, 2018]

[14] Stephens C. Huntsville Hospital Notifying 60 Patients of Possible Radiation Overdose from Brain Scan. 2009. Available from: http://blog.al.com/breaking/2009/12/huntsville_hospital_notifying.html [Accessed: November 10, 2017]

[15] Folven E. Patient Still Angry Over Radiation Overdoses. 2010. Available from: http://beverlypress.com/2010/10/patient-still-angry-over-radiation-overdoses/ [Accessed: November 10, 2017]

[16] Barnes E. California Governor Signs Medical Radiation Bill into Law. 2010. Available from: http://www.auntminnie.com/index.aspx?sec=ser&sub=def&pag=dis&ItemID=92208 [Accessed: November 10, 2017]

[17] Simons M. Brazil Gets Help on Radiation Accident. 1987. Available from: http://www.nytimes.com/1987/10/11/world/brazil-gets-help-on-radiation-accident.html [Accessed: November 10, 2017]

[18] Rojavin Y et al. Civilian nuclear incidents: An overview of historical, medical, and scientific aspects. Journal of Emergencies, Trauma, and Shock. 2011;**4**(2):260

[19] Ricks RC et al. Radiation accidents in the United States. In: Medical Management of Radiation Accidents. Boca Raton, Florida: CRC Press; 2001. pp. 173-178

[20] Commission, N.R. Loss of an Iridium-192 Source and Therapy Misadministration; November 16, 1992; Indiana, Pennsylvania: Indiana Regional Cancer Center. Nuclear Regulatory Commission; 1993

[21] Stawicki SP, Firstenberg MS. Introductory chapter: The decades long quest continues toward better, safer healthcare systems. In: Vignettes in Patient Safety. Vol. 1. Rijeka, Croatia: InTech; 2017

[22] Marks LB et al. The challenge of maximizing safety in radiation oncology. Practical Radiation Oncology. 2011;**1**(1):2-14

[23] Brandan M et al. Evaluation of diagnostic radiology services in five Latin American countries: Results for mammography. In: Radiological Protection of Patients in Diagnostic and Interventional Radiology, Nuclear Medicine and Radiotherapy. 2001. p. 151

[24] Semelka RC et al. The information imperative: Is it time for an informed consent process explaining the risks of medical radiation? Radiology. 2012;**262**(1):15-18

[25] Sodickson A et al. Recurrent CT, cumulative radiation exposure, and associated radiation-induced cancer risks from CT of adults. Radiology. 2009;**251**(1):175-184

[26] Pearce MS et al. Radiation exposure from CT scans in childhood and subsequent risk of leukaemia and brain tumours: A retrospective cohort study. The Lancet. 2012;**380**(9840): 499-505

[27] Wolbarst AB et al. Medical response to a major radiologic emergency: A primer for medical and public health practitioners. Radiology. 2010;**254**(3):660-677

[28] Chambers CE. Radiation Safety in the Cardiac Catheterization Laboratory. 2015. Available from: http://www.scai.org/Assets/46da1a06-6404-40e7-bd09-50e1ead03138/635863752010270000/2015fellows-06dec15-sun-am1600-1417-radiationsafety-chambers-pdf

[29] Wilson G. Overview of a radiation safety program in a district style medical environment. The Canadian Journal of Medical Radiation Technology. 2006;**37**(4):18-25

[30] O'dou TJ. Recycling and Reuse of Radioactive aterials; 2012

[31] World Health Organization. Organization and Implementation of a National Regulatory Infrastructure Governing Protection against Ionizing Radiation and the Safety of Radiation Sources. Interim Report for Comment. Food and Agriculture Organization of the United Nations; 1999

[32] Chambers E et al. Radiation safety program for the cardiac catheterization laboratory. Catheterization and Cardiovascular Interventions. 2011;**77**(4):546-556

[33] Jankowski CB. Radiation protection for nurses. Regulations and guidelines. The Journal of Nursing Administration. 1992;**22**(2):30-34

[34] Limacher MC et al. Radiation safety in the practice of cardiology. Journal of the American College of Cardiology. 1998;**31**(4):892-913

[35] Porter FT. Radiation Safety Annual Report 2012-2013

[36] Collins M. Clinical Reasoning in Image Guided Radiotherapy: A Multimethod Study. Sheffield Hallam University; 2018

[37] Trindade R, Paiva I. Radioactive Waste Management in Portugal. Disposal of Low Activity Radioactive Waste2004. p. 119

[38] Mercer DR. Prospectus on the Legislative Response to Medical Waste, A. Mo. L. Rev. Vol. 551990. p. 509

[39] Picano E. Informed consent and communication of risk from radiological and nuclear medicine examinations: How to escape from a communication inferno. BMJ [British Medical Journal]. 2004;**329**(7470):849

[40] Massachusetts General Hospital. Reducing Radiation Exposure. 2017. Available from: http://www.massgeneral.org/imaging/about/reducing_radiation_exposure.aspx [Accessed: December 8, 2017]

[41] FDA. Radiation-Emitting Products: Education and Communication. 2017. Available from: https://www.fda.gov/Radiation-EmittingProducts/RadiationSafety/RadiationDoseReduction/ucm299331.htm [Accessed: December 8, 2017]

[42] Mettler FA Jr. Communication of radiation benefits and risks in decision making: Communication on Children's imaging and computed tomography. Health Physics. 2011;**101**(5):589-590

[43] Image Wisely. Image Wisely: Radiation Safety in Adult Medical Imaging. 2017. Available from: http://www.imagewisely.org/ [Accessed: December 8, 2017]

[44] IAEA. Radiation Protection of Patients. 2017. Available from: https://www.iaea.org/resources/rpop [Accessed: December 8, 2017]

[45] Wikipedia. Federal Data Services Hub. 2019. Available from: https://en.wikipedia.org/wiki/Federal_Data_Services_Hub [Accessed: February 23, 2019]

[46] USNRC. The NRC: Who We Are And What We Do. 2018. Available from: https://www.nrc.gov/docs/ML1607/ML16076A366.pdf [Accessed: December 15, 2018]

[47] Lancellotti P et al. Expert consensus for multi-modality imaging evaluation of cardiovascular complications of radiotherapy in adults: A report from the European Association of Cardiovascular Imaging and the American Society of Echocardiography. European Heart Journal Cardiovascular Imaging. 2013;**14**(8):721-740

[48] Berthrong M. Pathologic changes secondary to radiation. World Journal of Surgery. 1986;**10**(2):155-170

[49] Kim S et al. Late gastrointestinal toxicities following radiation therapy for prostate cancer. European Urology. 2011;**60**(5):908-916

[50] Hull MC et al. Valvular dysfunction and carotid, subclavian, and coronary artery disease in survivors of Hodgkin lymphoma treated with radiation therapy. The Journal of the American Medical Association. 2003;**290**(21):2831-2837

[51] Leung TW et al. Radiation pneumonitis after selective internal radiation treatment with intraarterial 90yttrium-microspheres for inoperable hepatic tumors. International Journal of Radiation Oncology, Biology, Physics. 1995;**33**(4):919-924

[52] Monson JM et al. Clinical radiation pneumonitis and radiographic changes after thoracic radiation therapy for lung carcinoma. Cancer: Interdisciplinary International Journal of The American Cancer Society. 1998;**82**(5):842-850

[53] Hovdenak N, Fajardo LF, Hauer-Jensen M. Acute radiation proctitis: A sequential clinicopathologic study during pelvic radiotherapy. International Journal of Radiation Oncology, Biology, Physics. 2000;**48**(4):1111-1117

[54] Hamilton FE. Gastric ulcer following radiation. Archives of Surgery. 1947;**55**(4):394-399

[55] Roberts L. Radiation Accident Grips Goiania. JSTOR; 1987

[56] Turai I et al. Medical response to radiation incidents and radionuclear threats. The British Medical Journal. 2004;**328**(7439):568-572

[57] Liu Q et al. Clinical report of three cases of acute radiation sickness from a 60Co radiation accident in Henan province in China. Journal of Radiation Research. 2008;**49**(1):63-69

[58] Jaschke W et al. Radiation-induced skin injuries to patients: What the interventional radiologist needs to know. Cardiovascular and Interventional Radiology. 2017;**40**(8):1131-1140

[59] Seltzer SM et al. New national air-kerma-strength standards for 125I and 103Pd brachytherapy seeds. Journal of Research of the National Institute of Standards and Technology. 2003;**108**(5):337

[60] Linet MS, Pyo Kim K, Rajaraman P. Children's exposure to diagnostic medical radiation and cancer risk: Epidemiologic and dosimetric considerations. Pediatric Radiology. 2009;**39**(1):4-26

[61] Ohana O et al. Overuse of CT and MRI in paediatric emergency departments. The British Journal of Radiology. 2018;**91**(1085):20170434

[62] Niles LM et al. US emergency department trends in imaging for pediatric nontraumatic abdominal pain. Pediatrics. 2017;**140**(4)

[63] Hess EP et al. Trends in computed tomography utilization rates: A longitudinal practice-based study. Journal of Patient Safety. 2014;**10**(1):52-58

[64] Miglioretti DL et al. The use of computed tomography in pediatrics and the associated radiation exposure and estimated cancer risk. JAMA Pediatrics. 2013;**167**(8):700-707

[65] ACR. ACR Appropriateness Criteria: Radiation Dose Assessment Introduction. 2018. Available from: https://www.acr.org/-/media/ACR/Files/Appropriateness-Criteria/RadiationDoseAssessmentIntro.pdf [Accessed: December 15, 2018]

[66] Krestinina LY et al. Protracted radiation exposure and cancer mortality in the Techa River cohort. Radiation Research. 2005;**164**(5):602-611

[67] Huda W. Dose and image quality in CT. Pediatric Radiology. 2002;**32**(10):709-713

[68] Clarke R et al. 1990 Recommendations of the International Commission on Radiological Protection. Documents of the NRPB. Vol. 4(1)1993. pp. 1-5

[69] Valentin J. The 2007 Recommendations of the International Commission on Radiological Protection. Oxford: Elsevier; 2007

[70] Infante-Rivard C, Deadman JE. Maternal occupational exposure to extremely low frequency magnetic fields during pregnancy and childhood leukemia. Epidemiology. 2003; **14**(4):437-441

[71] Infante-Rivard C, Mathonnet G, Sinnett D. Risk of childhood leukemia associated with diagnostic irradiation and polymorphisms in DNA repair genes. Environmental Health Perspectives. 2000;**108**(6):495

[72] Shu XO et al. Diagnostic X-rays and ultrasound exposure and risk of childhood acute lymphoblastic leukemia by immunophenotype. Cancer Epidemiology, Biomarkers and Prevention. 2002;**11**(2):177-185

[73] Journy N et al. Predicted cancer risks induced by computed tomography examinations during childhood, by a quantitative risk assessment approach. Radiation and Environmental Biophysics. 2014;**53**(1):39-54

[74] Nguyen CP, Goodman LH. Fetal risk in diagnostic radiology. In: Seminars in Ultrasound, CT and MRI. Philadelphia, Pennsylvania: Elsevier; 2012

[75] Practice A.C.O.O. ACOG Committee Opinion Number 299, September 2004 (Replaces No. 158, September 1995). Guidelines for diagnostic imaging during pregnancy. Obstetrics and Gynecology. 2004;**104**(3):647

[76] Raptis CA et al. Imaging of trauma in the pregnant patient. Radiographics. 2014;**34**(3): 748-763

[77] Tirada N et al. Imaging pregnant and lactating patients. Radiographics. 2015;**35**(6): 1751-1765

[78] Manlove W et al. Role of MRI in Trauma in the Pregnant Patient, in MRI of Fetal and Maternal Diseases in Pregnancy. Cham, Switzerland: Springer; 2016. pp. 491-497

[79] Silviera ML et al. Complications related to endoscopic retrograde cholangiopancreatography: A comprehensive clinical review. Journal of Gastrointestinal and Liver Diseases. 2009;**18**(1):73-82

[80] Vock P. Clinical perspective on diagnostic X-ray examinations of pregnant patients–what to take into account. Physica Medica. 2017;**43**:165-171

[81] Tsuei BJ. Assessment of the pregnant trauma patient. Injury. 2006;**37**(5):367-373

[82] Sugrue M, Kolkman KA. Trauma during pregnancy. Australian Journal of Rural Health. 1999;**7**(2):82-84

[83] Raff GL et al. Radiation dose from cardiac computed tomography before and after implementation of radiation dose-reduction techniques. The Journal of the American Medical Association. 2009;**301**(22):2340-2348

[84] Kharbanda AB et al. Analysis of radiation dose to pediatric patients during computed tomography examinations. Academic Emergency Medicine. 2015;**22**(6):670-675

[85] Bordoli SJ et al. Radiation safety education in vascular surgery training. Journal of Vascular Surgery. 2014;**59**(3):860-864.e1

[86] Lekovic GP et al. Radiation exposure during endovascular procedures. Operative Neurosurgery. 2008;**63**(suppl_1):ONS81-ONS86

[87] Dindyal S, Rahman S, Kyriakides C. Review of the use of ionizing radiation in endovascular aneurysm repair. Angiology. 2015;**66**(7):607-612

[88] Harbaugh RE, Agarwal A. Training residents in endovascular neurosurgery. Neurosurgery. 2006;**59**(suppl_5):S3-277-S3-281

[89] Killewich LA et al. Factors Affecting Radiation Injury. Journal of Vascular Surgery. 2011;**53**:9S-14S

[90] Schanzer A et al. Vascular surgery training trends from 2001 to 2007: A substantial increase in total procedure volume is driven by escalating endovascular procedure volume and stable open procedure volume. Journal of Vascular Surgery. 2009;**49**(5):1339-1344

[91] Shah NB, Platt SL. ALARA: Is there a cause for alarm? Reducing radiation risks from computed tomography scanning in children. Current Opinion in Pediatrics. 2008;**20**(3):243-247

[92] Kuppermann N et al. Identification of children at very low risk of clinically-important brain injuries after head trauma: A prospective cohort study. The Lancet. 2009;**374**(9696):1160-1170

Chapter 5

The Anatomy of Medication Errors

Vasiliki Kapaki

Additional information is available at the end of the chapter

http://dx.doi.org/10.5772/intechopen.79778

Abstract

Medication errors constitute a category of errors that occur more frequently in healthcare units. They refer to every preventable event that may cause or lead to the inappropriate use of medicines or patient injury, during the therapeutic process. This type of events may be associated with professional practices, healthcare products, procedures, and systems including prescription, communication through instructions, drug labeling, packaging and nomenclature, reformulation, dissolution, distribution, administration, education, monitoring, and use. Classification and evaluation of medication errors according to their importance may constitute an important factor for process improvement in order to render the administration of medicines as safe as possible. The main categories of causes that lead to medication errors are those associated with the healthcare provider system, the healthcare professional, the pharmacy, and the scientific competence of the personnel. Technology has grown to be a constituent part of medicine these days. The appropriate technology is able to assist in increased efficiency, enhanced quality, and lessened costs. A few advantages that technology can supply are categorized as follows: the assisting of communication between clinicians; enhancing medication safety; decreasing potential medical errors and adverse events; rising access to medical information and encouraging patient-centered healthcare. The aim of this chapter is to provide a compendious literature review regarding the definition, the classification, the causes, and the main strategies for preventing medication errors.

Keywords: nursing error(s), medication error(s), definition, causes, classification, usage, adverse drug reaction(s) – adverse drug event(s), electronic medical record(s), patient safety

1. Introduction

The interest in the study of medication errors and adverse drug events has increased intensively after the publication of studies such as "To Err is Human: Building a Safer Health System" [1]

and "An Organization with a Memory" [2], which set a new milestone in patient safety. The administration of medicines constitutes a complex technique, which requires the participation of various healthcare professionals and takes place in a complex environment [3]. Nurses constitute a group of healthcare professionals who fill most of the prescriptions and spend 40% of their time in the hospital in order to administer pharmaceutical preparations to the patients [4]. Therefore, medication errors in nursing occur more frequently and have an impact not only on patient's health and safety but also on the healthcare system since prolonged hospitalization of patients generates additional costs, as a whole, for the healthcare system [5, 6].

For half a century, nurses learn the basic principles of the medication administration phase which are included in the following tenet: "appropriate patient, appropriate medicine, appropriate dosage, appropriate routes of administration, appropriate time." The implementation of the above tenet comprises an indicator of quality nursing care [7].

In 1981, Steel et al. discovered that more than half of the iatrogenic damages were associated with medication use. These consequences may vary from smaller or imperceptible to very serious and lethal [8].

The majority of studies regarding medication errors refer to hospital patients due to the fact that it is easier to perceive and register errors in hospitals than in the case of medication to be administered at home. It has been found that medication errors are mainly related to prescription, preparation, administration, and patient monitoring processes. Nurses' involvement in processes (prescription, preparation, and medicine administration as well as patient monitoring) other than prescription is instrumental, since the aforementioned processes constitute nursing actions performed on a daily basis [9].

The incidence of medication errors is just as high in developing countries as in the developed ones [10, 11]. Approximately 5% of the adverse drug events (ADEs) that could be ascribed to nurses administering medications to patients are likely to put patients' safety at risk [12]. Moreover, researches have shown that 1/3 of medication side effects (MSEs) result from medication errors [13]. The incidence of medication errors is higher in children than in adults, since dosages for children are estimated separately for each child depending on their age, weight, body surface, and clinical conditions. Additionally, the majority of medications for children are unlicensed and off-label [14–16].

According to the National Patient Safety Agency (NPSA), medication errors in the United Kingdom (UK) occur at all phases of the medication therapy: 16% in prescription, 18% in distribution, and 50% in medication administration. The equivalent rates in pediatrics range between 3–37% in prescription, 5–58% in distribution, 72–75% in administration, and 17–21% refer to clinical documentation errors. In a period of 8 years, 29 children have lost their lives due to medication errors in the UK [17]. Moreover, medication errors cause 1 of 131 outpatients and 1 of 854 inpatient deaths [1], and inpatient medication error rates are between 4.8% [18] and 5.3% [19]. It should be underlined that injury from medication errors is modest (0.9% of medication errors) [19]. Furthermore, the medications most usually involved with errors categorize insulin, opioid-containing analgesic, anticoagulant, amoxicillin-containing agent, and antihistamine/cold remedy [20].

It is estimated that medication errors cost the US healthcare system $77 million each year [21]. According to an older study, medication errors extend the hospitalization for an average of 4.6 days [22] and increase the cost at about $2000–2500 per patient [23].

http://dx.doi.org/10.5772/intechopen.79778

According to Allan and Barker, the purpose of examining medication errors is to measure the errors made in various healthcare organizations and the different error rates in relation to the implementation of different medication distribution systems, to identify the causes of these errors and to evaluate the practices employed for their prevention. The examination of all these parameters mainly aims at preventing the errors associated with medications for the protection of patients [24]. Originating a dependable area for all the categories of patients to be able to ask safety-related questions in a responsibility-free environment and urging, the errors and adverse events whenever they occur, revealed, along with the creation of layers of defense mechanisms (such as the use of computer based technical knowledge; uncomplicated images on wristbands and color coded alerts on handoff/sign-out materials) will all contribute to promote a genuine culture of safety on the inside of the healthcare system [25].

2. Summary of key points

Table 1 presents the most important points of the chapter concerning the medication errors.

Definitions	
Medication error	Any kind of error happening anywhere in the medication use procedure
Adverse drug event	An adverse result that can be ascribed to the action of a medicine
Epidemiology: statistics	
• Medication errors cause 1 of 131 outpatients and 1 of 854 inpatient deaths	
• Inpatient medication error rates are between 4.8 and 5.3%	
• Injury from medication errors is modest (0.9% of medication errors)	
• Medications most usually involved with errors are categorized as insulin, opioid-containing analgesic, anticoagulant, amoxicillin-containing agent, and antihistamine/cold remedy	
Risk factors	
Patient elements	Deterioration in renal or hepatic function, impaired cognition, comorbidities, and polypharmacy
Healthcare professionals' elements	Use of abbreviations, cognitive biases
Avoiding medication errors	
• Computerized physician order entry	
• Bar code-assisted administration	
• Enhanced medication labeling	
• Medication reconciliation	

Table 1. Medication errors: summary of key points.

3. Medication errors: terms and definitions

Meurier et al. defined nursing errors as "every action, decision or omission of a nurse which was evaluated as incorrect by more experienced colleagues and had adverse effects on patients" [26]. In 1954, the American Hospital Association (AHA) defined for the first time medication error as "the administration of the wrong medication, medication dosage, diagnostic or therapeutic substance, to the wrong patient or at the wrong time, or the failure to administer these substances at a given time or according to the prescription or what is considered as acceptable practice" [27].

The National Coordinating Council for Medication Error Reporting and Prevention (NCC MERP) defines medication errors as: "any preventable event, which may cause or lead to inappropriate use of medications or to patient injury, while medication therapy is under the control of a health care professional, patient or user of health services. Such events may be associated with professional practices, healthcare products, procedures and systems including prescription, communication via instructions, product labeling, packaging and nomenclature, reformulation, dissolution, distribution, administration, education, monitoring and use" [28].

Choo et al. defined medication error as "any error during the medication administration, regardless of whether they have consequences or not" [29]. According to an ethnographic study in 2003 regarding the impact and the significance of intravenous medication errors, intravenous medication errors are defined as: "a divergence between the preparation and administration of an intravenous medication and the medical prescription, the hospital strategy regarding intravenous administrations and the instructions of the manufacturer" [30].

The definitions of severity level for adverse drug events (ADEs) are presented in **Table 2** [31]. The relationship among medication errors, adverse drug events, and potential adverse drug events is illustrated in **Figure 1** [32].

Significant ADE	Happens if the event brings about symptoms that while substance to the patient creates little or no threat to the patient's life function. These ADEs could contain aggrandized or depressed laboratory test levels
	Examples of physical symptoms are categorized as sensation, physical tiredness, inability to defecate, muscle cramps, inability to sleep, headaches, and pedal edema
Serious ADE	Happens if the event brings about persistent alteration of life function. Moreover serious ADEs could contain aggrandized or depressed lab values that require medical intervention, exceptionally if they propose organ system dysfunction
	Examples of physical symptoms are categorized as a two-unit gastrointestinal bleed, a symptom requiring hospitalization, an altered mental status/excessive sedation, allergic reaction-shaking chills/fever, or symptomatic hypoglycemia
Life-threatening ADE	Happens if the event brings about symptoms or alterations that if not treated would put the patient at risk of death Life-threatening ADEs categorize laboratory values that are either aggrandized or depressed to the point that a crucial physiologic function is at risk of failure
	Examples of physical symptoms; patient transferred to ICU due to respiratory failure, cardiac arrest, and anaphylaxis

Table 2. Definition of severity level for adverse drug events (ADEs).

http://dx.doi.org/10.5772/intechopen.79778

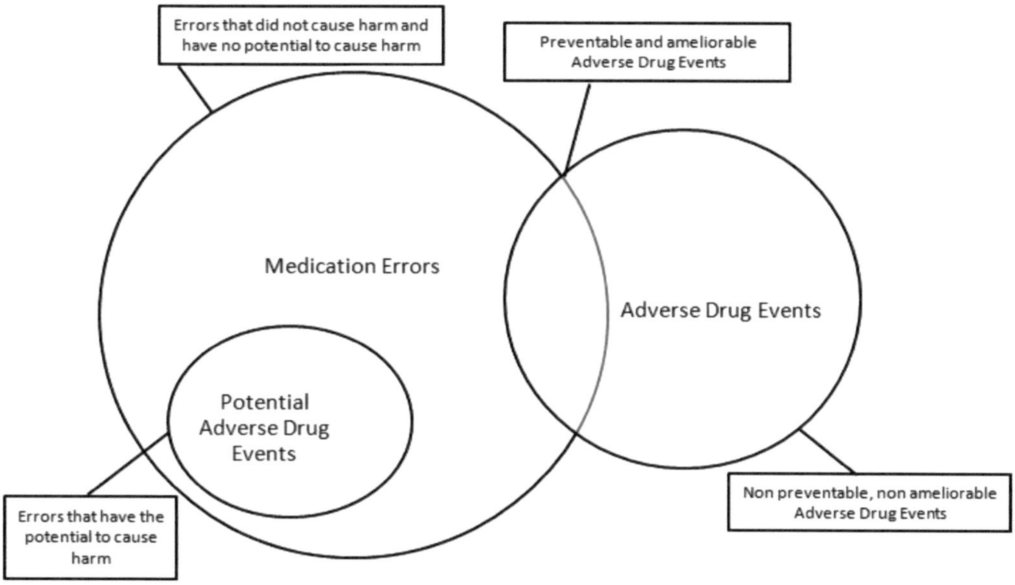

Figure 1. Relationship among medication errors, adverse drug events, and potential adverse drug events. Source: Gandhi et al. [32].

4. Classifications of medication errors

In 1960, Safren and Chapanis published the first study that documents the type of medication errors and classifies them into seven categories (wrong patient, wrong time, wrong dosage, omission of a dosage, administration of an extra dosage, wrong medicine, and wrong route of administration) [33].

Medication errors could be classified into two major categories: the ones that occur prior to medication administration, during the preparation, and upon medication administration [30].

i. Errors in preparation

   Medication preparation for the purpose of administration is a process that involves all these actions performed by nurses in order to reach the medication to patients ready for use. Some of the nursing medication errors upon preparation for hospitalization are [30, 34]:

- Errors in copying medical instructions
- Wrong method of preparation and drug dissolution
- Incorrect content of the reconstituted drug
- Incorrect selection of medication due to similar packaging
- Incorrect dosage due to miscalculations

ii. Errors in administration

Some of the most common errors in medication administration involve [30, 34]:

- Administering the wrong medication to the wrong patient
- Incorrect route of medication administration
- Incorrect rate of administration
- Incorrect method of administration
- Incorrect time of administration
- Repeated medication administration
- Medication administration without medical prescription
- Interruption of medication administration whereas it should be continued
- Continue medication administration against doctor's order to interrupt it
- No medication administration

The NCC MERP created an algorithm in order to classify medication errors into nine categories, based on the extent of the damage they may cause to the patient [35]:

iii. Conditions and events that may lead to an "error"

iv. An error that finally did not cause any damage to the patient

v. An error that occurred to a patient but did not cause any damage

vi. An error that occurred to a patient but required further monitoring or intervention in order to ensure that it did not cause any damage

vii. A temporary damage to the patient that requires intervention

viii. A temporary damage to the patient that requires initial or extended hospitalization

ix. Permanent disability of the patient

x. Intervention required in order to keep the patient alive

xi. Death of the patient

5. Assessment of medication errors

According to the literature, one of the main characteristics of medication errors is their severity. In 1986, the El Dorado Medical Centre in Tucson, Arizona, developed a tool for the evaluation of medication errors, the so-called El Dorado Medication Error Tool (EDMET). This tool is objective, is uncomplicated to use, and defines clearly the four parameters, which are related to the severity of medication errors. These parameters are associated with the type of errors (i.e., wrong time, route, date, dosage, preparation, rate of administration, extra dosage, omission of a dosage), the route of administration (i.e., intravenous, intramuscular, oral, etc.), the classification of drugs according to a particular list that includes drugs with serious side effects in case of an error (i.e., heparin, digoxin, potassium), and the time between the medication error and the identification thereof. The last parameter constitutes an important role regarding patient's outcome, since it determines early or belated initiation of interventions that will prevent or reverse adverse consequences. Moreover, the abovementioned parameters are further categorized and rated each time depending on the situation. Finally, the total score depends on whether the patient has stated any allergies to a certain medication. This tool is particularly easy to use; it is designed to be accurate and reliable, and it has been used by the center in order to evaluate the severity of errors on the one hand and to determine further interventions by nursing stuff on the other. According to these data, classification and evaluation of medication errors depending on their severity may constitute an important tool for the improvement of processes in order to make medication administration as safe as possible [36].

6. Etiology of medication errors

Safren and Chapanis were the first to classify the causes of medication errors into 10 categories (not following any audit process, illegible medical instructions, errors in copying instructions, errors in classifying instructions, errors in calculating the dosage, improvisations, wrong medication labels, patient assignment to two nurses at the same time, poor oral communication, and more). Other criteria for the documentation involve the status of the person that made the mistake (student or worker), the nursing department where the error occurred, the time of day, and the severity of the patient's condition [33].

Wakefield et al. classified the causes of medication errors into five categories this time [37]. The first category refers to the causes associated with the system (regular interruptions of nurses upon administering the medications, regular changes of nurses, simultaneous administration of medication for all the patients, poor authentication of patient's identity). The second category refers to the causes associated with the healthcare professional (failure to transpose instructions into the medication cards, poor communication between nurses regarding medication dosages that have not been administered, errors in copying instructions, noncompliance with the medication administration processes). This category also includes poor compliance of the healthcare professional with hospital policies and procedures, fragmentary personal experiences of the nurses [38], and memory lapses [39].

Other categories refer to causes related to doctors (illegible, unclear instructions, frequent changes of the instructions), pharmacies (imprecise medication dosage and administration or wrong dosages), and the adequate knowledge of the staff (inadequate knowledge regarding adverse reactions of medications, poor access to Manuals of Pharmacology). Apart from these five categories of errors, it is worth referring to the causes that have been mentioned by other authors including incorrect mathematical calculations; poor dosage adjustment, in order to prevent liver and kidney damages; inability to obtain a proper medical history that may also include possible allergies to medication preparations; and inability to prevent synergistic effects between two or more drugs and to further convey this information to health professionals [40, 41]. Part of medication errors is largely attributable to lack of relevant information regarding the new technologies, such as the function of medical drug delivery pumps [39].

Other causes of medication errors are associated with working conditions at the sites where medical products are produced, i.e., lighting conditions, noise, packaging, and nomenclature for medical products, i.e., medications with similar names, distribution and storage processes, and processes and protocols specified in every agency [42–45].

The NCC MERP documented 10 basic factors that influence medication use process and are frequently associated with the causes of medication errors. These 10 factors involve information related to the medical history of the patient; medications; communication between healthcare professionals, in order to convey information regarding medications; nomenclature and packaging of medication preparations; storage, safekeeping, and standardization of medication; acquisition, use, and monitoring of medication devices; environmental factors; competence and education of the staff and the patient; and quality and risk management processes [46].

7. Consequences of medication errors

The consequences of medication errors vary; the instance, however, that the error becomes apparent and the immediate action for the prevention or reversal of adverse events are of critical importance. The impact of medication errors on patients who are admitted in intensive care units (ICU) is more serious, since most of the times these patients receive a considerable amount of medications and they are often characterized by impaired capacity to adapt to the consequences of such errors (due to organ failure, possible immunosuppressant, poor communication, etc.). The consequences of medication errors may be associated with extended hospitalization and application of additional interventions, or they may be life-threatening for the life of the patient and may even lead to death [11].

In a study of Bates et al., every error related to drugs was responsible for an average of 2.2 more days of stay in the ICU [47]. In another study, despite the fact that no lethal errors were observed, 26 of them were potentially threatening to patients' lives, whereas 55 of them were considered important [48]. Moreover, a study of Calabrese et al. did not observe any lethal errors, but five of them contributed to the need for increased monitoring of the patient and two of them led to the implementation of an appropriate intervention [49]. On the contrary, Flaatten and Hevroy found that one error led to the death of a patient; five (5.7%) were evaluated as important, whereas twenty two (25%) contributed to the implementation of an appropriate intervention [50]. Finally, in a study of Rothschild et al. (2005), 120 AE were reported,

14 of which (11.6%) were threatening for the life of patients and 2 (1.6%) of them were lethal, whereas 24 (11%) of the 222 errors which were reported were evaluated as potentially threatening for the life of patients [51].

8. Prevention of medication errors

The use of technology contributes to the improvement of the quality of the services provided and maximizes the protection and safety of patients against eventual errors and events throughout healthcare provision. Intranet installation as well as the use of personal computers in healthcare provision units contributes to the implementation of automated (computerized) systems for the writing of medical instructions, therefore eliminating errors attributable to illegible handwritings [52].

It also minimizes errors that occur while copying instructions on medication cards and prevents questions and misinterpretations, since every prescription includes mandatory fields that must be completed, such as route and time of administration as well as the precise dosage. Using special software for pharmacology, nurses can also be informed about possible allergies or side effects from incompatible medications every time they check on a patient's medical record. The placement of barcodes on every medication as well as the placement of identification wristbands for every patient upon admission to the hospital may decrease errors associated with inappropriate administration of medications with similar packaging and the administration of the wrong medication to the wrong patient. Using a wireless device at the time of hospitalization, nurses are able to monitor the administration of the appropriate medication preparation to the correct patient in the appropriate dosage using the appropriate route [53].

The use of "smart" infusion pumps for intravenous medication administration and more specifically for the administration of unsafe preparations, such as heparin or insulin, predetermines the infusion rate and provides security alarms. Such pumps have been used for several years in specialized departments, such as ICU. The rapid technological development contributed to further improvement of the existing pumps by customizing them and giving the healthcare professional the ability to enter information, such as possible allergic reactions, for every patient or install a software with pharmacology data [54].

Additionally, nurses should ensure the correctness of their actions not only during the preparation but also during the execution of hospitalization, thereby eliminating any external interference. Preparation of hospitalization is also advised as well as dissolution of intravenous preparations, at a separate, individual space and not in the room, where patients may pose various questions to the nurse. Moreover, patients' escorts should not be in the wards during hospitalization, so that it is quite and the nurses can concentrate on the administration of medications without anything distracting their attention [54].

Last but not least, the medication errors may also be prevented by simplifying nursing actions, by developing and establishing guidelines and protocols that will be followed systematically during the preparation and the administration of medications. Yet it is imperative to ensure the proper staffing of every health institution with nursing staff, in order to increase the ratio of nurses to patients.

9. Electronic medical records and medication errors

Electronic medical records (EMRs) constitute the only reliable implementation of medical, nursing, and laboratory work, since they have limited errors and improved productivity, and the medical decisions of the past provided essential support regarding the administration of medication treatment and the detection of abnormalities in laboratory examinations. They have also improved significantly the quality of the health services provided. The complete development and implementation of EMRs further require the development of an integrated information system [55, 56].

Some of the most important benefits of EMRs regarding medications are [55–60]:

- **i.** Elimination of medical errors
- **ii.** Physician productivity improvement
- **iii.** Minimization of cost
- **iv.** Encouragement of greater cooperation between sectors
- **v.** Quality improvement of the provided services
- **vi.** Systematic organization and nursing documentation through the use of legible medical records
- **vii.** Prevention of medication errors
- **viii.** Minimization of the time that is required for written procedures
- **ix.** Avoiding duplication of information required for the daily planning of the interventions
- **x.** Communication through the use of a common language
- **xi.** Easy and quick search and data recovery aiming at information but also with the potential of immediate information processing and grouping
- **xii.** Faster and more efficient communication and arrangement of procedures that require cross-sectorial cooperation
- **xiii.** Valid economic analysis of hospitalization costs for every patient based on the registered interventions, laboratory exams, medications, and materials
- **xiv.** Statistical process and evaluation of clinical nursing applications
- **xv.** Possibility of data and folder filing with simultaneous space saving
- **xvi.** Access of nurses to electronic libraries
- **xvii.** Familiarity and active participation of nurses in the information society and the circulation of knowledge
- **xviii.** Improvement of information quality (clear, inclusive, reliable, always available)

xix. Direct dissemination of common information at every level of information management (order, supply, administration, implementation of intervention, charge)

xx. Complete workflow automation

xxi. Process definition and implementation at section level and cross-sectorial cooperation

xxii. Increase of individual and group efficiency and effectiveness

xxiii. Possibility of direct and effective intervention of the competent institution in cases of any discrepancies in the management of medication products, materials, and laboratory exams

xxiv. Ability to monitor the availability of every type of pharmaceutical products

xxv. Ability to monitor physical and electronic stocks of every department

xxvi. Positive impact on the financial management of the insurance funds and the hospital due to a decrease of fictitious overconsumption of medications.

10. Clinical vignette

Louisa Bright, a 77-year-old, used to wake up at night with a difficulty in breathing with wheezing. Her doctor diagnosed her with asthma and gave her a prescription with albuterol, a bronchodilator. Two days later, Mrs. Bright was admitted to the coronary care unit (CCU) of a hospital with a heart attack. In his letter to the team leader of the medical department, the cardiologist reported that Mrs. Bright's doctor had made a wrong diagnosis regarding the wheezing of congestive heart failure and had prescribed a wrong treatment for asthma. The cardiologist reported that the therapy could have accelerated heart attack.

11. Conclusion

Errors in the administration of medication treatment constitute a consequential causation of morbidity and mortality, yet it could be an unclear and underappreciated understanding. A medication error is any error that happens in the medication use procedure. It has been assessed by the IOM that medication errors bring about 1 of 131 outpatient and 1 of 854 inpatient deaths. Medication elements (e.g., sounding names, below normal-level therapeutic index), patient elements (e.g., unsatisfactory renal or hepatic function, impaired knowledge, polypharmacy), and healthcare professional elements (e.g., use of abbreviations, perceptual biases) are able to bring about faster medication errors. Frequent effects faced by physicians after medication errors can be categorized as loss of patient trust, civil actions, criminal charges, and medical board discipline. Procedures to prevent medication errors from happening (e.g., use of information technology, better drug labeling, and medication reconciliation) have been used with inconsistent satisfactory outcome.

If an error or an adverse drug event is realized, most patients anticipate disclosure that is at a suitable time, given in person, and accompanied with an apology and attempt to prevent future adverse drug events and errors. Learning more about medication errors may improve healthcare professionals' capacity to make available cautious healthcare to their patients. Future research should concentrate on recognizing the errors and adverse drug events that most usually cause patient injury. Furthermore, a better knowledge in what manner of information technology, labeling, medication reconciliation, and improved care transitions decrease medication errors and adverse drug events is needed. A concentration of easy-to-use and cheap techniques for medication error lowering will probably have the greatest influence.

Acknowledgements

The author did not get any dedicated funding for the specific manuscript.

Competing interests

The author affirms that she has no competing interests.

Abbreviations

ADEs	adverse drug events
AEs	adverse events
AHA	American Hospital Association
CCU	coronary care unit
EDMET	El Dorado medication error tool
EMRs	electronic medical records
ICUs	intensive care units
MSEs	medication side effects
NCC MERP	National Coordinating Council for Medication Error Reporting and Prevention
NPSA	National Patient Safety Agency
UK	United Kingdom
US	United States

Author details

Vasiliki Kapaki

Address all correspondence to: vkapaki2005@gmail.com

Health Policy Institute, Athens, Greece

References

[1] Institute of Medicine (US) Committee on Quality of Health Care in America. In: Kohn LT, Corrigan JM, Donaldson MS, editors. To Err is Human: Building a Safer Health System. Washington (DC): National Academies Press (US); 2000

[2] Donaldson L. An organisation with a memory. Clinical Medicine. 2002;**2**(5):452-457

[3] Lilford R, Stirling S, Maillard N. Citation classics in patient safety research: An invitation to contribute to an online bibliography. Quality & Safety in Health Care. 2006;**15**(5):311-313

[4] Armitage G, Knapman H. Adverse events in drug administration: A literature review. Journal of Nursing Management. 2003;**11**(2):130-140

[5] Lehmann CU, Conner KG, Cox JM. Preventing provider errors: Online total parenteral nutrition calculator. Pediatrics. 2004;**113**(4):748-753

[6] Mrayyan MT, Shishani K, Al-Faouri I. Rate, causes and reporting of medication errors in Jordan: Nurses' perspectives. Journal of Nursing Management. 2007;**15**(6):659-670

[7] Rolen M. The nurse's role in accident prevention. Nursing Outlook. 1955;**3**(11):588-590

[8] Steel K et al. Iatrogenic illness on a general medical service at a university hospital. 1981. Quality & Safety in Health Care. 2004;**13**(1):76-80

[9] Mangino PD. Role of the pharmacist in reducing medication errors. Journal of Surgical Oncology. 2004;**88**(3):189-194

[10] McCarthy AM, Kelly MW, Reed D. Medication administration practices of school nurses. The Journal of School Health. 2000;**70**(9):371-376

[11] Mihailidis A, Krones L, Boger J. Assistive computing devices: A pilot study to explore nurses' preferences and needs. Computers, Informatics, Nursing. 2006;**24**(6):328-336

[12] Hughes RG, Ortiz E. Medication errors: Why they happen, and how they can be prevented. Journal of Infusion Nursing. 2005;**28**(2 Suppl):14-24

[13] Hashemi F. Response ethics to nursing errors. Journal of Medical Ethics and History of Medicine. 2007;**4**:31-46

[14] Cuzzolin L, Atzei A, Fanos V. Off-label and unlicensed prescribing for newborns and children in different settings: A review of the literature and a consideration about drug safety. Expert Opinion on Drug Safety. 2006;**5**(5):703-718

[15] Lindell-Osuagwu L et al. Off-label and unlicensed drug prescribing in three paediatric wards in Finland and review of the international literature. Journal of Clinical Pharmacy and Therapeutics. 2009;**34**(3):277-287

[16] Pandolfini C, Bonati M. A literature review on off-label drug use in children. European Journal of Pediatrics. 2005;**164**(9):552-558

[17] Thomas AN, Panchagnula U. Medication-related patient safety incidents in critical care: A review of reports to the UK National Patient Safety Agency. Anaesthesia. 2008; **63**(7):726-733

[18] Jimenez Munioz AB et al. Medication error prevalence. International Journal of Health Care Quality Assurance. 2010;**23**(3):328-338

[19] Bates DW et al. Incidence of adverse drug events and potential adverse drug events. Implications for prevention. ADE Prevention Study Group. Journal of the American Medical Association. 1995;**274**(1):29-34

[20] Budnitz DS et al. National surveillance of emergency department visits for outpatient adverse drug events. Journal of the American Medical Association. 2006;**296**(15):1858-1866

[21] Tang FI et al. Nurses relate the contributing factors involved in medication errors. Journal of Clinical Nursing. 2007;**16**(3):447-457

[22] Keohane CA, Bates DW. Medication safety. Obstetrics and Gynecology Clinics of North America. 2008;**35**(1):37-52 (viii)

[23] Bates DW et al. Relationship between medication errors and adverse drug events. Journal of General Internal Medicine. 1995;**10**(4):199-205

[24] Allan EL, Barker KN. Fundamentals of medication error research. American Journal of Hospital Pharmacy. 1990;**47**(3):555-571

[25] Thomas AN, Belser D, Rabenold S, Bamgbelu OO, Mandalapu A, Pipestone M, A Mira A-E, Baxter R. Wrong Patient, Wrong Drug: An Unfortunate Confluence of Events in Vignettes in Patient Safety: Michael S. Firstenberg, IntechOpen; 2017. DOI: 10.5772/intechopen.69168. Available from: https://www.intechopen.com/books/vignettes-in-patient-safety-volume-1/wrong-patient-wrong-drug-an-unfortunate-confluence-of-events

[26] Meurier CE, Vincent CA, Parmar DG. Learning from errors in nursing practice. Journal of Advanced Nursing. 1997;**26**(1):111-119

[27] American Hospital Association. Hospital Safety Manual for Use by Hospital Administrators and Department Heads. Chicago: American Hospital Association; 1954

[28] United States Pharmacopeia (USP). USP medication error reporting program. [updated on 2008 Dec 1]. Available from: http://www.usp.org/patientSafety/reporting/mer.html

[29] Choo J, Hutchinson A, Bucknall T. Nurses' role in medication safety. Journal of Nursing Management. 2010;**18**(7):853-861

[30] Taxis K, Barber N. Ethnographic study of incidence and severity of intravenous drug errors. British Medical Journal. 2003;**326**(7391):684

[31] Sawarkar A et al. Adverse drug events caused by serious medication administration errors. BMJ Quality and Safety. 2012;**21**(11):933-938

[32] Gandhi R. Management of the treatment experienced patient. The Hopkins HIV Report. 2000;**12**(2):1, 8-9, 15

[33] Safren MA, Chapanis A. A critical incident study of hospital medication errors. Hospitals. 1960;**34**:32-34; passim

[34] Wright K. Do calculation errors by nurses cause medication errors in clinical practice? A literature review. Nurse Education Today. 2010;**30**(1):85-97

[35] Hartwig SC, Denger SD, Schneider PJ. Severity-indexed, incident report-based medication error-reporting program. American Journal of Hospital Pharmacy. 1991;**48**(12): 2611-2616

[36] Cobb MD. Evaluating medication errors. The Journal of Nursing Administration. 1986; **16**(4):41-44

[37] Wakefield BJ et al. Nurses' perceptions of why medication administration errors occur. Medsurg Nursing. 1998;**7**(1):39-44

[38] Fuqua RA, Stevens KR. What we know about medication errors: A literature review. Journal of Nursing Quality Assurance. 1988;**3**(1):1-17

[39] Leape LL et al. Systems analysis of adverse drug events. ADE Prevention Study Group. Journal of the American Medical Association. 1995;**274**(1):35-43

[40] LaPointe NM, Jollis JG. Medication errors in hospitalized cardiovascular patients. Archives of Internal Medicine. 2003;**163**(12):1461-1466

[41] Lesar TS, Briceland L, Stein DS. Factors related to errors in medication prescribing. Journal of the American Medical Association. 1997;**277**(4):312-317

[42] Gladstone J. Drug administration errors: A study into the factors underlying the occurrence and reporting of drug errors in a district general hospital. Journal of Advanced Nursing. 1995;**22**(4):628-637

[43] O'Shea E. Factors contributing to medication errors: A literature review. Journal of Clinical Nursing. 1999;**8**(5):496-504

[44] Schlossberg E. 16 Safeguards against medication errors. Hospitals. 1958;**32**(19):62; passim

[45] Walters JA. Nurses' perceptions of reportable medication errors and factors that contribute to their occurrence. Applied Nursing Research. 1992;**5**(2):86-88

[46] Cousins DD, Heath WM. The National Coordinating Council for Medication Error Reporting and Prevention: Promoting patient safety and quality through innovation and leadership. Joint Commission Journal on Quality and Patient Safety. 2008;**34**(12):700-702

[47] Bates DW et al. The costs of adverse drug events in hospitalized patients. Adverse Drug Events Prevention Study Group. Journal of the American Medical Association. 1997;**277**(4):307-311

[48] Tissot E et al. Medication errors at the administration stage in an intensive care unit. Intensive Care Medicine. 1999;**25**(4):353-359

[49] Calabrese AD et al. Medication administration errors in adult patients in the ICU. Intensive Care Medicine. 2001;**27**(10):1592-1598

[50] Flaatten H, Hevroy O. Errors in the intensive care unit (ICU). Experiences with an anonymous registration. Acta Anaesthesiologica Scandinavica. 1999;**43**(6):614-617

[51] Rothschild JM et al. The Critical Care Safety Study: The incidence and nature of adverse events and serious medical errors in intensive care. Critical Care Medicine. 2005;**33**(8):1694-1700

[52] Gibson T. Nurses and medication error: A discursive reading of the literature. Nursing Inquiry. 2001;**8**(2):108-117

[53] Crawford M, Mullan J, Vanderveen T. Technology and safe medication administration. The American Journal of Nursing. 2005;**105**(3 Suppl):37-41; quiz 4851

[54] Vanderveen T. How IV safety systems have prevented medication errors. Journal of Infusion Nursing. 2005;**28**:40-41

[55] Nelson SD et al. Link between prescriptions and the electronic health record. American Journal of Health-System Pharmacy. 2018;**75**(11 Suppl 2):S29-S34

[56] Hron JD et al. Electronic medication reconciliation and medication errors. International Journal for Quality in Health Care. 2015;**27**(4):314-319

[57] Fernando B et al. Approaches to recording drug allergies in electronic health records: Qualitative study. PLoS One. 2014;**9**(4):e93047

[58] Zhao J et al. Predictive modeling of structured electronic health records for adverse drug event detection. BMC Medical Informatics and Decision Making. 2015;**15**(Suppl 4):S1

[59] Czaja AS et al. Electronic health record (EHR) based postmarketing surveillance of adverse events associated with pediatric off-label medication use: A case study of short-acting beta-2 agonists and arrhythmias. Pharmacoepidemiol Drug Safety. 2018

[60] Nemeth LS, Wessell AM. Improving medication safety in primary care using electronic health records. Journal of Patient Safety. 2010;**6**(4):238-243

Chapter 6

Combating Alarm Fatigue: The Quest for More Accurate and Safer Clinical Monitoring Equipment

James Nguyen, Kendra Davis,
Giuseppe Guglielmello and Stanislaw P. Stawicki

Additional information is available at the end of the chapter

http://dx.doi.org/10.5772/intechopen.84783

Abstract

As the demand for health-care services continues to increase, clinically efficient and cost-effective patient monitoring takes on a critically important role. Key considerations inherent to this area of concern include patient safety, reliability, ease of use, and cost containment. Unfortunately, even the most modern patient monitoring systems carry significant drawbacks that limit their effectiveness and/or applicability. Major opportunities for improvement in both equipment design and monitor utilization have been identified, including the presence of excessive false and nuisance alarms. When poorly optimized, clinical alarm activity can affect patient safety and may have a negative impact on care providers, leading to inappropriate alarm response time due to the so-called alarm fatigue (AF). Ultimately, consequences of AF include missed alerts of clinical significance, with substantial risk for patient harm and potentially fatal outcomes. Targeted quality improvement initiatives and staff training, as well as the proactive incorporation of technological improvements, are the best approaches to address key barriers to the optimal utilization of clinical alarms, AF reduction, better patient care, and improved provider job satisfaction.

Keywords: alarm fatigue, clinical alarms, clinical monitoring, monitoring equipment, patient safety

1. Introduction

Highly reliable, precise, user-friendly, and cost-effective clinical alarm systems are critical to efficient functioning of health-care facilities [1–3]. Despite tremendous progress over the past few decades, the "perfect solution" remains elusive, with focus being placed primarily on clinical indications and appropriateness of use for the existing equipment and monitoring frameworks [3–6]. Beyond the concept of "false alarm," suboptimal implementation of clinical monitoring systems can have much more profound and potentially dangerous consequences [7–9]. One such consequence, and the primary topic of this chapter, is the phenomenon of alarm fatigue (AF). It is defined as the decrease of clinician response caused by excessive alarms, sensory overload, and desensitization, in addition to other occupational and environmental variables [9–11]. Among contributing factors are also high staff workload, long shift hours, and work environments with high noise levels, all of which contribute to the "desensitization effect" associated with AF [10, 12].

Hospital patient care units tend to be high-paced and potentially unpredictable environments, with complex workflows. Multiple simultaneous interactions between patients, families, and health-care staff may create an added element of chaos [13, 14]. To help nurses and other staff cope with their many responsibilities, various audible and visual alerts have been implemented to prompt immediate response and clinical assessment of patients [15]. These alerts are relayed from patient monitoring devices, which provide continuous flow of vital sign data with a high degree of sensitivity. The advanced technology used in these surveillance systems has provided a significant amount of physiological data at low cost while being particularly helpful by facilitating the monitoring of critically ill patients to identify deviations of vital signs (e.g., heart rate, respiratory rate, blood pressure, and pulse oximetry) from normal ranges [16]. However, when various clinical alarm systems are superimposed on the need for constant vigilance in the setting of highly challenging and often chaotic environment of the typical clinical unit, the stage is set for the emergence of AF and other forms of cognitive lapses [17–19].

The prevalence of various monitoring modalities has increased significantly, with most health-care institutions utilizing some broadly defined combination of different alarm systems. As the use of these systems became more widespread, a major flaw became evident: the excessive amount of triggered alarms was contributing to unintended consequences, both in terms of patient outcomes and staff fatigue/dissatisfaction [8, 20, 21]. The high rate of nonactionable alarms, where immediate action is not required on the behalf of clinicians, was especially problematic [22]. In fact, the increasing frequency of "false alarms" has a significant desensitization effect on hospital staff, whereby some alarms may be erroneously "dismissed by assumption" as being "noncritical" [23]. This desensitization leads to both increased response times and decreased, or even lack of, clinician response. In the setting of a busy hospital, it is commonplace to hear constant chimes and beeps, each coming from different machines and indicating different "alarm conditions" (**Figure 1**). It should be more of an expectation that clinicians become desensitized to extraneous stimuli given the constant sensory bombardment coupled with the need for vigilance and differential interpretation of each alarm [25, 26]. When further compounded by heavy clinical workloads and long shifts, it becomes a matter of "statistical probability" before a critical alarm is missed [27–29]. Given the effect of this potentially dangerous phenomenon on both quality and safety of patient care, closer scrutiny of AF and related concepts is warranted. In this chapter, we will present a vignette-based discussion outlining fairly typical AF scenarios. Opportunities for improvement, including equipment, personnel, and systems-based considerations, will then be provided.

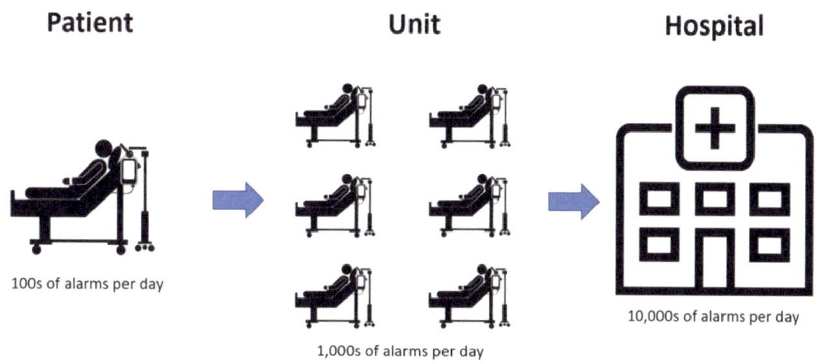

Figure 1. Conceptual model for daily observed alarms at a typical acute care hospital. Data shown in proportion to different scales, from individual patient to entire institution, showing the true magnitude of the problem (source: Ref. [24]).

2. Primary research methods

For the purposes of this chapter, the authors performed a thorough literature search using PubMed, Google Scholar™, and Bioline International. Primary search terms included "alarm fatigue," "health-care alarms," "patient monitoring," "provider burnout," as well as secondary terms consisting of various combinations of primary search terms. From over 47,000 unique search results, we distilled 73 most pertinent references immediately relevant to this document. Finally, additional sources that were cited across our primary search results were added, for a total of 101 references included in the final manuscript.

3. Patient monitoring: different types and modalities

A diverse number of patient monitors are widely used across various health-care settings [30–32]. When employed correctly, they provide potentially valuable, actionable, and real-time information about a patient's clinical status. Different monitoring devices are intended to measure different parameters, potentially allowing for rapid assessment of a patient. This is especially relevant in the context of the current discussion of AF and more specifically the domain of alarm trigger accuracy [32, 33]. As clinical monitoring becomes more sophisticated and better integrated, remote (off-site) implementations also become possible [34–36]. The subsequent discussion will outline major types of monitoring equipment and alarms, including ventilation/oxygenation, hemodynamic, and pressure point alert systems.

3.1. Ventilation/oxygenation alarms

In general, primary ventilation/oxygenation alarms (VOA) include capnography and pulse oximetry, respectively. More broadly, respiratory parameter monitoring indicates the patient's oxygen saturation, respiratory rate, and end-tidal carbon dioxide [33, 37]. The use of VOA has been particularly important for critically ill patients who require mechanical ventilatory support. In such applications, the monitor is designed to be exquisitely sensitive to detect even the slightest changes in a patient's oxygenation or ventilation status [38]. As demonstrated in *Clinical Vignette #1* later in the chapter, an alarm may be triggered following the detection of a very small respiratory parameter "excursion," regardless of its clinical significance or magnitude of the observed change in the patient's actual clinical status. In this context, apnea and minute volume warnings are among the most common alarms triggered, with majority of such occurrences deemed clinically irrelevant upon further interrogation [39]. Moreover, many VOA triggers can be attributed to artifactual sources (e.g., patient movement, interruption of blood flow by inflating blood pressure cuff, and even atmospheric pressure variations) [37]. Thus, providers should be educated accordingly to ensure that the above considerations are appropriately factored into final clinical determinations and decisions.

3.2. Hemodynamic alarms

Hemodynamic alarms (HA) monitor a variety of parameters, of which the most common ones include heart rate, systolic/diastolic/mean blood pressure, and various other intravascular pressure measurements via both invasive and noninvasive approaches [37, 40]. Hemodynamic monitoring has become a useful tool for the bedside assessment of patients in a number of clinical scenarios, from routine telemetry applications to advanced intravascular catheter utilization. There is some degree of predictability based on measured parameters, especially when trend determination and volume responsiveness are being considered [41, 42]. Hemodynamic monitors are particularly important in the setting of an unstable (or potentially unstable) patient, similar to the one described in *Clinical Vignette #3* later in the chapter. In such capacity, HAs can help facilitate rapid intervention and prompt correction of emergent issues. Still, HAs are far from perfect, with significant shortcomings in their discriminatory capabilities. More specifically, HAs are unable to identify a patient as "stable" or "unstable," especially when physiologic compensatory processes mask any underlying instability or in the setting of rapid change in hemodynamic status [43]. Thus, when using any particular monitoring modality, there is no substitute for an astute clinician who is able to effectively correlate HA findings with the clinical reality [44–46].

3.3. Bed and chair pressure sensors

Bed and chair pressure sensor (BCPS) alarms are utilized across many hospitals and other health-care facilities to help reduce mechanical falls among patients who experience ambulatory or balance difficulties [47, 48]. Falls typically occur as patients attempt to mobilize and/or ambulate without the required assistance of trained health-care staff [49]. Consequently, the use of BCPS alarms serves to alert staff—typically by a pressure-sensitive mechanism—when a patient attempts to move from a bed or chair without assistance. However, the weight-sensitive pads are easily triggered by very slight patient movement, resulting in a significant number of false alarms [50, 51]. This challenge was readily apparent in *Clinical Vignette #3* later in the chapter, as the majority of BCPS alerts were likely due to the patient merely shifting slightly in the bed, and not by an actual attempt to independently mobilize and/or ambulate.

Unfortunately, the one true positive alarm became lost in "a sea of false negatives." The practicality of BCPS alarms is also diminished by the inability of staff members to immediately assess/respond to the triggered alarm. Instances have been noted in which the alarm signal is transmitted after the event already transpired, as patients tend to fall immediately upon leaving the bed or chair [52].

In summary, the above-referenced monitor/alarm types have become an important part of the modern health-care fabric. Despite their ubiquitous use and great potential for constructive and practical clinical application, each type of device carries inherent flaws that providers must be aware of. Detailed knowledge of the risk-benefit equation associated with each device and clinical alarm type is important not only for patient safety but also required to help improve the quality and accuracy of the next generation of monitoring devices.

4. Patient monitor alarm design

Patient monitors are designed to have high sensitivity to predefined changes in various measured parameters, including vital signs, respiratory/ventilator status, and patient movements. However, the major drawback associated with high alarm sensitivity is the poor specificity and inherently disproportionate number of nonactionable (or nonclinical) alarms triggered [22, 53, 54]. Depending on the specific alarm and clinical setting, the estimated in range of "false positives" may be as high as 80–99% of all triggered alarms [8]. Broadly speaking, nonactionable alarms can be categorized as false alarms, nuisance alarms, and technical alarms (**Figure 1**). To elaborate further, false alarms occur in the absence of an actual patient or system trigger and typically result from a measurement artifact [55]. Technical alarms mandate the provider to attend to some operational aspect of the monitoring system, such as when readjustment of monitor leads/sensors is required [21]. Nuisance alarms are defined as clinically insignificant alarms that may interfere with patient care [10]. In aggregate, these nonactionable alarms are a major cause of the overall desensitization of hospital staff that may ultimately result in AF (**Figure 2**).

Furthermore, to be effective, the alarms transmitted by monitoring systems must trigger some degree of cognitive response in health-care providers. This equates to introducing stress and the need for constant vigilance, both of which further heighten the risk of AF [56, 57]. When multiple clinical competing priorities collide, it becomes increasingly difficult for a provider to proactively address all ongoing problems, thus forcing them to resort to only partially addressing acute issues while at the same time disrupting other (parallel) activities due to multitasking [58–61]. Consequently, an ideal alarm should be perfectly audible and easily recognized by health-care providers working within the patient care unit [8], while at the same time minimizing the amount of stress imposed on the responding clinical staff.

The increasingly complex environment of modern health-care systems has led to several important considerations regarding the practical application of monitoring systems. For example, space-related issues deserve special mention, with overly crowded clinical units creating an abundance of alarm-related stimuli and geographically larger clinical units

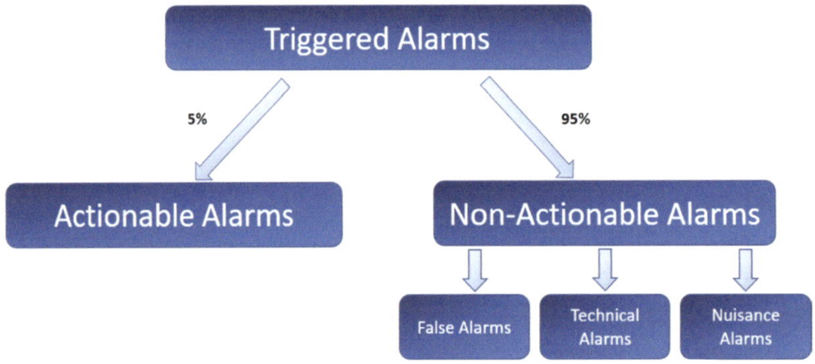

Figure 2. Schematic representation of the classification of alarm types triggered by various patient monitoring systems, including both actionable and nonactionable alerts (source: Ruskin [8]; Gorges [66]; and Tsien [67]).

presenting a barrier to prompt patient access. Elevated acuity and high patient throughput are also important considerations in this context [62].

Furthermore, technological advancements facilitated the development of increasingly sophisticated alarm systems, with novel features designed to decrease the nuisance factor of the alert mechanism while preserving the level of overall clinical vigilance [63, 64]. These are intended to provide a range of alarm tones that allow care providers to easily identify and prioritize alarms, typically as high, medium, or low priority. However, the implementation of such systems (e.g., IEC 60601-1-8 standard) has presented challenges in terms of recognizability of melodic alarm tones. More specifically, nurses found it difficult to accurately identify all of the melodic tones signifying high-priority alarms, in addition to the potential for confusion between certain alarm pairs [65]. An example of such phenomenon is presented in *Clinical Vignette #1* below, where two sets of tones were too difficult for the nurse to readily differentiate, rendering the alarm feature ineffective. Consequently, it is important for systems to have some degree of built-in learnability and flexible discriminative ability, with continued refinement, development, and testing of each clinical alarm, both alone and in tandem with other competing alarms [65]. Without exception, any observed deficits in patient monitor effectiveness and/or safety should prompt an immediate critical evaluation of both technical and clinical aspects of its implementation and function.

5. Clinical Vignettes

5.1. *Clinical Vignette #1*: 62-year-old female presenting with chronic obstructive pulmonary disease (COPD) exacerbation

A 62-year-old female was admitted to the local hospital 5 days ago due to chronic obstructive pulmonary disease (COPD) exacerbation. She was diagnosed with COPD several years prior and remained stable with no history of exacerbations until 1 week ago when she developed a progressively worsening cough. Soon after her symptoms worsened, she began to feel shortness of breath that was not relieved by rest. At this point, her family insisted she go to the

http://dx.doi.org/10.5772/intechopen.84783

hospital for evaluation. Upon arriving in the emergency department, short-acting bronchodilators and oral corticosteroids were administered with only mild symptomatic improvement. Given the patient's dyspnea at rest, as well as decreased oxygen saturation of 86%, she was admitted to the pulmonology unit. Supplemental oxygen and intravenous corticosteroids were administered.

At admission, continuous pulse oximetry monitoring was started. The patient's hypoxemia seemed to improve slightly over the next 4 days, with oxygen saturation climbing to 88–90% range. Still, the patient's ventilatory monitor sent alarm signals to the hospital staff several times an hour due to high respiratory rate and episodic oxygen desaturations. Alarm signals were transmitted as either a single low tone (respiratory rate) or a double alarm (desaturations), alternating between low and medium tones. The difference of alarm tone indicated the range in which the patient's oxygen saturation was measured, but the assigned night-shift nurse found the tones to be too difficult to distinguish and would routinely just perform an in-person check of the saturation level upon entering the room. Throughout the first two nights, the same nurse responded to the alarms in a timely fashion, only to find the patient stable and with no signs of acute distress. Assuming that alarms are unlikely to represent any actionable clinical events, the same nurse then began to silence the sounds and began checking on the patient hourly. In the early morning hours of the fourth day, the nurse silenced the alarm once again, intending to assess the patient once the remainder of her rounding routine was completed. When the nurse finally came to the patient's room an hour later, she found the patient unresponsive and cyanotic. A rapid assessment showed an oxygen saturation of 79%. The patient was immediately intubated, transferred to intensive care unit, and mechanical ventilation was initiated.

5.2. *Clinical Vignette* #2: 65-year-old male transferred to inpatient unit following a total knee arthroplasty

A 65-year-old male with a history of osteoarthritis of the right knee and refractory pain underwent preoperative evaluation by an orthopedic surgeon. Given his adequate performance status and lack of comorbidities, the patient was determined to be a suitable candidate for total right knee arthroplasty. The surgical procedure was uneventful, with appropriate antibiotic and venous thrombosis prophylaxis administered perioperatively. Following a brief recovery in the postanesthesia care unit, the patient was transferred to the inpatient floor with expected discharge within 5 days postsurgery. Due to the nature of his surgery and apparent fall risk, the patient's room was fitted with weight-sensitive bed and chair alarms. During the first 3 days, he remained relatively sedated due to the frequent administration of pain medications. However, as the patient began to regain strength, his analgesia regimen was tapered. On day 4, the concurrent increase in patient's movement began to trigger his bed monitor to the point where the on-call nurse was receiving nearly constant alarm notifications. Multiple times, the nurse entered to assess the patient only to find him resting comfortably without apparent attempt to leave his bed. Later that night, after leaving the patient's room, the nurse was unexpectedly assigned to three additional patients due to an unplanned absence of a coworker. As the nurse hurried to assess the new patients, the bed monitor transmitted yet another alarm signal. Annoyed by the repeated negative alarms, the nurse disabled the alerts from the bed monitor, intending to check in after tending to her newly assigned patients. When she finally returned to the patient's room, she found him sprawled on the floor and writhing in pain. The patient, emboldened by his rapid recovery, had attempted to ambulate to the bathroom without assistance and lost his balance in the process. The intense pain prevented him from reaching the call button on the hospital bed, so he was forced to lie on the floor in pain for approximately 1 h. A subsequent skeletal survey revealed a left hip fracture, which required additional surgery, prolonged hospital stay, and the need for inpatient rehabilitation stay due to temporary disability involving bilateral lower extremities (e.g., right knee arthroplasty and left hip injury).

5.3. *Clinical Vignette #3*: 71-year-old male with history of multiple myeloma admitted for right lower extremity swelling associated with minor pain

A 71-year-old male with a history of multiple myeloma was admitted to the urgent care center after noticing sudden onset of right lower extremity swelling associated with minor pain. The patient began induction therapy for multiple myeloma approximately 1 year prior, achieving adequate disease control. He was subsequently transitioned to maintenance treatment, which he continued for the past 6 months. Evaluation in the urgent care center with venous duplex studies revealed a deep venous thrombosis (DVT). Because of the patient's established history of malignancy, the triage clinician opted for hospital admission and therapeutic anticoagulation. While being transferred to the inpatient unit, unfractionated heparin anticoagulation was started. Per standard protocol, monitoring equipment was hastily fitted to the patient for noninvasive measurement of his blood pressure and heart rate. Overnight, the patient remained stable, with some resolution of lower extremity of pain despite persistent swelling. The on-call physician assessed the patient during morning rounds and ordered to repeat venous duplex for the afternoon to evaluate for resolution/progression of the DVT. Of note, throughout the night and into the morning hours, the patient's hemodynamic monitor had been sending intermittent alarm signals. With the first few alarms, the charge nurse promptly responded and quickly assessed the patient for any signs of instability or distress. However, as the shift progressed, the nurse increasingly dismissed repeated signals as "false alarms" due to a recurring pattern of mildly elevated blood pressure and heart rate secondary to episodic extremity pain. Because the inpatient unit continued to be understaffed during the morning shift, the charge nurse decided to disable the patient's repeated monitor alarms after the patient was assessed during morning rounds and found not to have any acute issues. It was hoped that this decision would eliminate the distraction of the nuisance alarms. However, during the patient's routine afternoon assessment, the rounding physician noted cold and diaphoretic extremities with markedly increased swelling. Interrogation of the monitor system revealed progressive bradycardia and hypotension over the past hour. An emergency CT angiogram showed a massive pulmonary embolism, prompting immediate thrombolytic therapy and patient transfer to intensive care. Despite aggressive management, the patient's shock became refractory, culminating in his death several hours later.

5.4. Summation of Clinical Vignettes: finding common threads

The three hypothetical clinical scenarios outlined above share a common theme: dedicated monitoring systems implemented to ensure early detection of clinical deterioration and thus patient safety were utilized either ineffectively or incorrectly. In all three vignettes, a confluence of factors (environment, patient, medical personnel) subsequently led to AF and then adverse patient outcomes. In the following sections, we will further discuss the phenomenon of alarm fatigue, focusing on its impact on daily clinical practice.

6. Alarm fatigue

After the general introduction of AF earlier in the chapter, the authors will now discuss this important concept in greater detail. The phenomenon of AF is multifaceted and includes increased clinician response time with simultaneous decreased response rate that is mainly attributed to excessive stimuli from clinical alarms [8]. Depending on patient acuity and clinical monitoring requirements, typical bedside health-care personnel may be exposed to as many as 1000 alarms during a single shift, of which as many as 95% can be nonactionable and thus do not require immediate clinical determination [8, 66, 67]. Given the multitude of clinical alarms, a provider has to sort through during a typical hospital shift, there will be a natural tendency to potentially dismiss certain alarms as insignificant through rationalization. This phenomenon is described in the literature as the natural human behavioral reaction to "deprioritize signals" that have often been proven to be either false or misleading. Thus, staff may begin reflexively disabling or silencing alarm systems, which could effectively mask other alarms that may be clinically significant [68, 69]. To some extent, this behavioral pattern was seen in all three *Clinical Vignettes,* where the actionable alarm was masked by the vast number of nonactionable alarms that preceded it. Ultimately, the resulting delay in response or inadequate response puts patient safety at risk and may result in morbidity and/or mortality [70, 71]. Technologically advanced physiologic monitors bring a lot of promise, both in terms of earlier and more sensitive detection of patient deterioration (or other clinically significant event); however, the sensory overload and desensitization associated with AF will likely continue to present a major opportunity for improvement.

Certain other factors have been implicated in the increased incidence and severity of alarm fatigue, including greater staff workload, higher patient acuity, and the complexity of the modern health-care environment [10]. Nurses serve as key frontline staff in most clinical settings and play a pivotal role in overseeing patient care and monitoring. Moreover, nurses are subject to significant occupational stress that can be attributed to multiple causes, including heavy workloads [72]. This stress, as outlined in previous sections of this chapter, certainly influences AF by forcing nurses to instantaneously adjust their work activities (and priorities) according to perceived importance of near constant clinical alarm activity. Our *Clinical Vignette #2* illustrated the difficult task of ongoing patient triage, with the nurse having to prioritize between the three newly admitted patients and all of her other assigned patients. This constant need for clinical vigilance and prioritization is potentially disruptive to typical workflow, especially when high task complexity is involved. It can also contribute to the development of burnout [73]. Nurses have expressed the internal conflict between having to ignore the constant alarms simply to maintain sufficient focus to finish their routine tasks [74]. It is not surprising that increasing workload or task complexity has been associated with both suboptimal job performance and inconsistent alarm response [10]. Furthermore, the

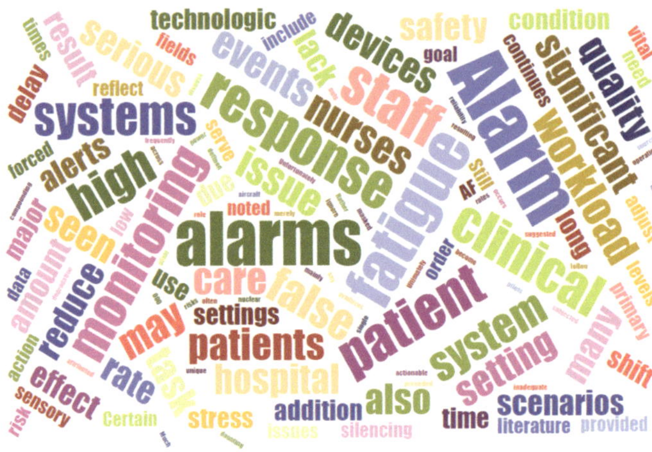

Figure 3. The word cloud demonstrating the multifaceted phenomenon of alarm fatigue.

effort of acknowledging, evaluating, and responding to an alarm significantly increases the overall time commitment and workload of the nurses, which further perpetuates the trend of decreased alarm response and task performance [8].

Because multiple factors contribute to AF, many existing models struggle to fully account for (and address) clinician behavioral patterns seen with AF [75]. At the same time, it should be noted that AF is not unique to clinicians. In fact, a similar phenomenon has also been seen among human operators utilizing automated monitoring systems, such as aircraft pilots and nuclear power plant operators. The excessive number of alarm activations leads to the tendency of operators to ignore alerts, particularly when the monitoring system produces a high rate of false alarms or alerts [75]. For these operational environments, it has also been suggested that increased primary and secondary task workloads have a compounding effect on alarm response degradation that may occur in the setting of low alarm system reliability [76]. Similar to the clinical setting, AF can be associated with serious safety risks and represents a similar barrier to the practical application of automated monitoring systems in other fields (**Figure 3**).

7. Potential outcomes of alarm fatigue

Significant percentage of nonactionable alarms in the typical modern clinical environment can lead to the development (and subsequent habituation) of AF. As previously mentioned, AF can be characterized by alarm desensitization, mistrust of alert accuracy/utility, and delay of caregiver response (or even lack thereof). Commonly seen reactions to AF include the deactivation and silencing of systems or adjustment of alarm parameters to decrease the number of alarms. Such reactive behaviors have the potential to result in missed critical alarms, leading to patient morbidity or even mortality. In fact, patient safety considerations associated with AF are among the top items of Emergency Care Research (ECRI)

Institute's Health Technology Hazards list [77, 78]. The subject of AF has been extensively studied, primarily due to its high prevalence across essentially all health-care settings. The underreporting of alarm-related events has been recognized as a challenge, and it should be noted that recorded incidents likely reflect only a small proportion of actual events. Available records from the Joint Commission's Sentinel Event Database show 98 alarm-related occurrences between January 2009 and June 2012 (**Figure 4**). Of these reported events, several common alarm system issues (**Figure 5**) were directly connected to events leading to injury or death (**Table 1**) [79].

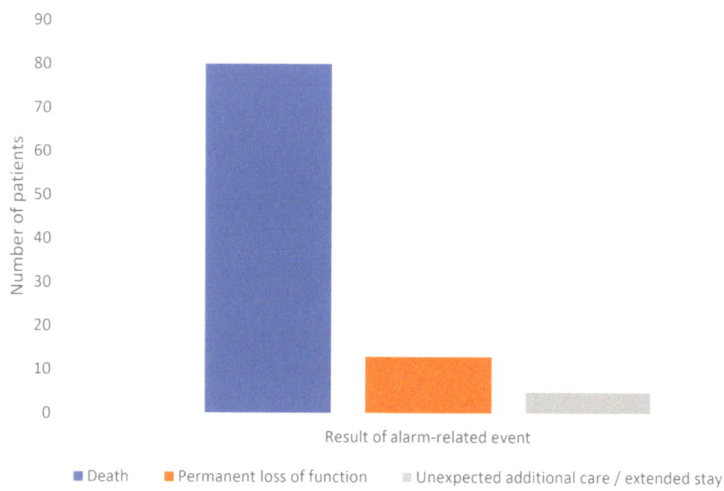

Figure 4. Alarm-related events and subsequent results from January 2009 to June 2012 (source: Joint Commission's Sentinel Event Database).

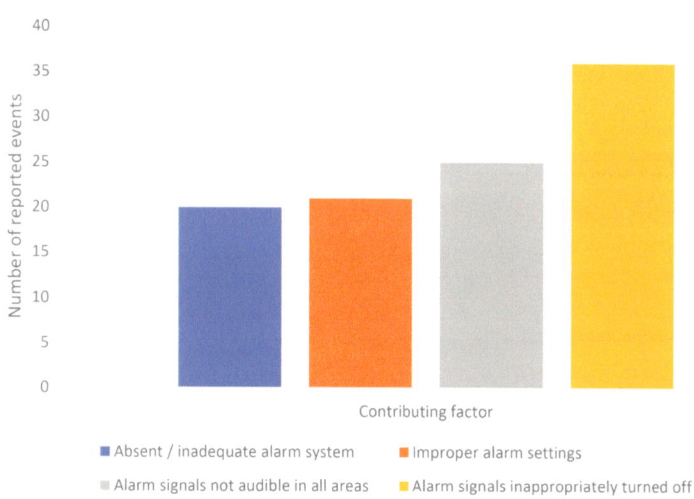

Figure 5. Major contributing factors of alarm-related events (source: Joint Commission's Sentinel Event Database).

Event
Falls
Delays in treatment
Delays in ventilator use
Medication errors
Source: Ref. [24].

Table 1. Common alarm-related events leading to injuries or deaths.

Additionally, the US Food and Drug Administration's Manufacturer and User Facility Device Experience (MAUDE) database has identified 566 alarm-related patient deaths between January 2005 and June 2010 [79]. Reports detailing alarm-related events have prompted thorough investigation into AF and possible strategies to address this important phenomenon in the clinical setting.

8. Quality improvement

Considering the potential for very serious clinical consequences of AF, quality improvement measures have been proposed to help reduce both nonactionable alarm occurrences and the incidence of AF. Successful quality improvement projects must address multiple facets of the overall problem, including root causes that lead to AF (**Figure 6**). For example, poor usability and lack of user-centered devices have the potential for elevating clinical personnel stress levels, creating unnecessary workload and interjecting workflow inefficiencies into an already tense environment [81].

Potential solutions for reducing the incidence of AF include multipronged approaches consisting of staff education, equipment (hardware and software) enhancements, and implementation of more efficient clinical protocols or guidelines [82–84]. From an educational perspective,

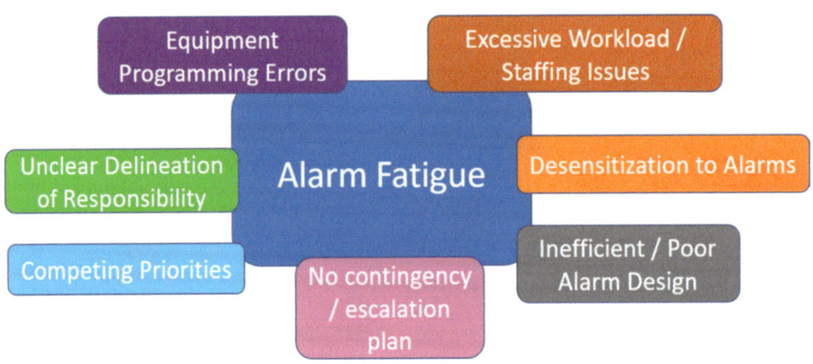

Figure 6. The different aspects of alarm fatigue that can be addressed through different quality improvement approaches (source: Ref. [80]).

it is important to ensure adequate staff education, equipment training, and closer team collaboration to improve patient safety within the existing framework [8, 85]. In addition to staff education, hospital policies have been developed and implemented to more clearly define which staff members are able to change alarm settings, as well as how such changes should be made and documented. Many of these polices have also delegated the responsibility of performing clinical alarm monitoring rounds to a staff member in order to allow for continued review of the application of patient monitoring systems [86–88].

To address the issues of staff workload, two potential approaches have been proposed. The first approach consists of secondary notification systems. The second option involves the use of dedicated staff to oversee alarms. A secondary notification system involves a specialized network interface that algorithmically facilitates the decision process regarding which alarms will be further communicated or escalated to pertinent downstream clinical staff. Further, this system would also enable the automatic escalation of an alert to another clinician, should the primary recipient fail to acknowledge the alarm within a designated timeframe. The use of staff to oversee alarms, while an expensive option, can give additional support to care providers in the form of dedicated personnel whose responsibility is to continuously monitor patient data trends and alarms from a central station [58].

No matter the solution, all the quality improvement processes require a multidisciplinary approach to address the causes and effects of AF. Only through collaborative efforts can substantial change be accomplished to reduce the number of alarm-related events in health care. In addition to the quality improvement measures taken by hospitals, technological advances have also led to more efficient and practical application of patient monitors in the clinical setting. These advances are directed at the reduction of nonactionable alarms with the goal of decreasing the alarm desensitization associated with AF. The importance of adequate information technology support, including better device designs, must be emphasized. As increasingly efficient and complex monitoring equipment is introduced into the clinical realm, certain phenomena, such as the emergence of "unpredictable code," may adversely affect computer performance (including the ability to effectively recognize important data patterns) and lead to clinical alerts being missed despite the fact that alert-specific data were clearly and provably present [89].

9. Technological advances in patient monitors

In general, clinical monitoring is based on a careful balance between sensitivity and specificity of alarm signal recognition, as well as the associated threshold setting required to trigger "alert condition" [90, 91]. Increasing monitor sensitivity helps ensure that truly significant events are not missed, primarily using single-parameter alarms and default thresholds [8]. However, as a trade-off this increases the incidence of nuisance alarms that are nonactionable. This issue may be remedied by the development of "smart alarm systems" that use algorithmic approaches to evaluate multiple parameters prior to determining whether the detected change is truly critical, and only then sending an alert to the operator [15]. This improvement in device specificity would result in significantly fewer false alarms and therefore reduce

System	Description	Application
Rule-based expert systems	Application of expert knowledge from a compiled database to new context and simulation of expert decisions	Development of a highly specific patient monitor system with electronic access to data available in a multichannel patient monitor and data management system to detect cardiac disturbances [37, 96]
Neural networks	Utilization of artificial neural networks to predict disease presence based on advanced information	Development of neuronal network used to detect myocardial infarction early on in patients admitted for chest pain [37, 97]
Fuzzy logic	Diffuse processing of exact data that does not indicate an explicit conclusion	Development of a monitor system able to diagnose simulated cardiac arrest via evaluation of EKG, capnography, and arterial blood pressure [37, 98]
Bayesian networks	System used for the estimation of event occurrence based on causal probabilistic networks	Application of system for decision support in cardiac event detection [37, 99]

Source: Schmid et al. [37].

Table 2. Applications of artificial intelligence in the development of intensive care monitoring.

AF. At the same time, the challenges of "unpredictable code" and "interrupted or corrupt data" have been noted and may represent an important safety issue due to the potential for missing data or data misinterpretation, especially when using memory-intensive applications on devices that are continually operating for prolonged periods of time [89, 92–95].

The ideal patient monitor would have high sensitivity, as well as high negative predictive value for life-threatening clinical scenarios. This would result in excellent "event detection rate" while reducing the number of false and nuisance alarms. Still, any improvement of sensitivity/negative predicative value for monitors must be accompanied by corresponding adjustment to specificity/positive predictive value, ensuring that clinically significant events are captured efficiently [33]. The accomplishment of the above goals may be possible using the application of artificial intelligence (AI) in monitoring systems, wherein AI would be incorporated into logic-based, decision-making systems. The ultimate goal would be the development of clinical monitoring capabilities that reflect and mirror human cognitive/decision-making processes [37]. In the context of this chapter's *Clinical Vignettes*, the application of such AI-based systems might be helpful in minimizing the number of nonactionable alarms, thus reducing the subsequent AF associated with adverse clinical events. So far, the utilization of AI has been explored in several different applications (**Table 2**).

10. Conclusion

Given the proliferation of advanced monitoring equipment, AF continues to be a major patient safety issue across modern health-care systems. While technological advances show great promise in improving patient care, significant barriers to more optimal implementations exist, including the ongoing struggle to balance the need for high sensitivity versus the excessive number nonactionable clinical alarms. The high frequency of clinical alerts, especially when combined with heavy clinical workload, is known to have negative effects of hospital staff, including alarm desensitization and subsequent delay and/or lack of caregiver response. The resultant AF poses a serious risk to patient safety and has been associated with significant adverse events, including the need for additional or prolonged hospital care, excess attributable morbidity, and even mortality. Prevention of AF requires a multipronged approach consisting of quality improvement measures, staff training, better equipment management (e.g., monitor threshold adjustments) to reduce false alarms, and focus on optimizing staff workload.

Author details

James Nguyen[1], Kendra Davis[2], Giuseppe Guglielmello[3] and Stanislaw P. Stawicki[4]*

*Address all correspondence to: stawicki.ace@gmail.com

1 Medical School of Temple University/St. Luke's University Health Network, Bethlehem, Pennsylvania, USA

2 Department of Surgery, Division of Acute Care Surgery, Traumatology and Surgical Critical Care, St. Luke's University Health Network, Bethlehem, Pennsylvania, USA

3 Department of Medicine, Section of Pulmonary and Critical Care Medicine, St. Luke's University Health Network, Bethlehem, Pennsylvania, USA

4 Department of Research and Innovation, St. Luke's University Health Network, Bethlehem, Pennsylvania, USA

References

[1] Kesselheim AS et al. Clinical decision support systems could be modified to reduce 'alert fatigue' while still minimizing the risk of litigation. Health Affairs. 2011;**30**(12):2310-2317

[2] Oppenheim MI et al. Design of a clinical alert system to facilitate development, testing, maintenance, and user-specific notification. In: Proceedings of the AMIA Symposium. Bethesda, Maryland: American Medical Informatics Association; 2000

[3] Konkani A, Oakley B, Bauld TJ. Reducing hospital noise: A review of medical device alarm management. Biomedical Instrumentation & Technology. 2012;**46**(6):478-487

[4] Edholm K et al. Decrease in inpatient telemetry utilization through a system-wide electronic health record change and a multifaceted hospitalist intervention. Journal of hospital medicine. Aug 2018;**13**(8):531-536

[5] Chen EH. Appropriate use of telemetry monitoring in hospitalized patients. Current Emergency and Hospital Medicine Reports. 2014;**2**(1):52-56

[6] Ivonye CC et al. Is telemetry overused? Is it as helpful as thought? Cleveland Clinic Journal of Medicine. 2009;**76**:369

[7] Lynn LA, Curry JP. Patterns of unexpected in-hospital deaths: A root cause analysis. Patient Safety in Surgery. 2011;**5**(1):3

[8] Ruskin KJ, Hueske-Kraus D. Alarm fatigue: Impacts on patient safety. Current Opinion in Anesthesiology. 2015;**28**(6):685-690

[9] Solet JM, Barach PR. Managing alarm fatigue in cardiac care. Progress in Pediatric Cardiology. 2012;**33**(1):85-90

[10] Cvach M. Monitor alarm fatigue: An integrative review. Biomedical Instrumentation & Technology. 2012;**46**(4):268-277

[11] West P, Abbott P. Alarm fatigue: A concept analysis. On-Line Journal of Nursing Informatics. 2014;**18**(2):1-5

[12] Deb S. Definition of Alarm Fatigue and its Influence on Staff Performance. Bozeman, Montana: Montana State University-Bozeman, College of Engineering; 2014

[13] Atkinson D. Nursing Observation and Assessment of Patients in the Acute Medical Unit. Salford, UK: University of Salford.; 2013

[14] Enerlan-Aas G. Coordinating Resources in Hospital: Complex Workflow. Tromsø, Norway: Universitetet i Tromsø; 2008

[15] Guardia-Labar LM et al. Alarm fatigue: The human-system interface. Clinical Nurse Specialist. 2014;**28**(3):135-137

[16] Wilken M et al. Alarm fatigue: Causes and effects. Studies in Health Technology and Informatics. 2017;**243**:107-111

[17] Patrick RA. TeamSTEPPS Training and Vital Signs Chart to Improve Situational Monitoring for Clinical Deterioration. Lexington, Kentucky; 2017

[18] Guastello SJ et al. Catastrophe models for cognitive workload and fatigue in a vigilance dual task. Human Factors. 2014;**56**(4):737-751

[19] Bellwood P. Qualitative Study of Technology-Induced Errors in Healthcare Organizations. Victoria, British Columbia, Canada: University of Victoria; 2013

[20] Harrison MI, Koppel R, Bar-Lev S. Unintended consequences of information technologies in health care—An interactive sociotechnical analysis. Journal of the American Medical Informatics Association. 2007;**14**(5):542-549

[21] Welch J. An evidence-based approach to reduce nuisance alarms and alarm fatigue. Biomedical Instrumentation & Technology. 2011;**45**(s1):46-52

[22] Cipriano A et al. Reducing telemetry use while improving patient outcomes: University health network experience with the implementation of oximetry-based monitoring system. International Journal of Academic Medicine. 2018;**4**(2):112-118

[23] Pyke JB. Analysis of Inpatient Surveillance Data for Automated Classification of Deterioration. Hanover, New Hampshire: Dartmouth College; 2012

[56] Weinger MB, Smith NT. Vigilance, Alarms, and Integrated Monitoring Systems. Anesthesia Equipment: Principles and Applications. Malvern, PA: Mosby Year Book; 1993. pp. 350-384

[57] Barach P, Sanchez JA. Redesigning hospital alarms for reliable and safe care. In: Surgical Patient Care. Cham, Switzerland: Springer; 2017. pp. 263-275

[58] Karnik A, Bonafide CP. A framework for reducing alarm fatigue on pediatric inpatient units. Hospital Pediatrics. 2015;**5**(3):160-163

[59] Kalisch BJ, Aebersold M. Interruptions and multitasking in nursing care. The Joint Commission Journal on Quality and Patient Safety. 2010;**36**(3):126-132

[60] Nolan TW. System changes to improve patient safety. BMJ: British Medical Journal. 2000;**320**(7237):771

[61] Laxmisan A et al. The multitasking clinician: Decision-making and cognitive demand during and after team handoffs in emergency care. International Journal of Medical Informatics. 2007;**76**(11-12):801-811

[62] Hussain M, Dewey J, Weibel N. Reducing alarm fatigue: exploring decision structures, risks, and design. EAI Endorsed Transactions on Pervasive Health and Technology. 2017;**3**:1-4

[63] Moffatt-Bruce SD, Huerta T. From ideas to institute for the design of environments aligned for patient safety (IDEA4PS): The reality of research and the keys to making it work. International Journal of Academic Medicine. 2016;**2**(3):2

[64] Edworthy J. Medical audible alarms: A review. Journal of the American Medical Informatics Association. 2012;**20**(3):584-589

[65] Lacherez P, Seah EL, Sanderson P. Overlapping melodic alarms are almost indiscriminable. Human Factors. 2007;**49**(4):637-645

[66] Gorges M, Markewitz BA, Westenskow DR. Improving alarm performance in the medical intensive care unit using delays and clinical context. Anesthesia and Analgesia. 2009;**108**(5):1546-1552

[67] Tsien CL, Fackler JC. Poor prognosis for existing monitors in the intensive care unit. Critical Care Medicine. 1997;**25**(4):614-619

[68] Phillips J, Barnsteiner JH. Clinical alarms: Improving efficiency and effectiveness. Critical Care Nursing Quarterly. 2005;**28**(4):317-323

[69] Varpio L et al. The helpful or hindering effects of in-hospital patient monitor alarms on nurses: A qualitative analysis. CIN: Computers, Informatics, Nursing. 2012;**30**(4):210-217

[70] Bridi AC, Louro TQ, da Silva RC. Clinical alarms in intensive care: Implications of alarm fatigue for the safety of patients. Revista Latino-Americana de Enfermagem. 2014;**22**(6):1034-1040

[71] Edworthy J. Alarms are still a problem! Anaesthesia. 2013;**68**(8):791-794

[72] Happell B et al. Nurses and stress: Recognizing causes and seeking solutions. Journal of Nursing Management. 2013;**21**(4):638-647

[73] Tolentino JC et al. What's new in academic medicine: Can we effectively address the burnout epidemic in healthcare? International Journal of Academic Medicine. 2017;**3**(3):1

[74] Solvoll T, Arntsen H, Hartvigsen G. Alarm fatigue vs user expectations regarding context-aware alarm handling in hospital environments using CallMeSmart. Studies in Health Technology and Informatics. 2017;**241**:159-164

[75] Bailey JM. The implications of probability matching for clinician response to vital sign alarms: A theoretical study of alarm fatigue. Ergonomics. 2015;**58**(9):1487-1495

[76] Bliss JP, Dunn MC. Behavioural implications of alarm mistrust as a function of task workload. Ergonomics. 2000;**43**(9):1283-1300

[77] Allan SH et al. Data-driven implementation of alarm reduction interventions in a cardiovascular surgical ICU. Joint Commission Journal on Quality and Patient Safety. 2017;**43**(2):62-70

[78] ECRI. Alarm Safety Resource Center: Guidance and Tools to Help Healthcare Facilities Improve Alarm Safety. 2018. Available from: https://www.ecri.org/re-center/Pages/Alarms.aspx

[79] The Joint Commission Medical device alarm safety in hospitals. Sentinel Event Alert. 8 April 2013;(50):1. https://www.ncbi.nlm.nih.gov/pubmed/23767076

[80] ECRI Institute. Top 10 Technology Hazards for 2012. 5 March 2019. Available online at: http://www.marylandpatientsafety.org/html/education/2012/handouts/documents/Top%2010%20Technology%20Hazards%20for%202012%20Article.pdf

[81] Sowan AK et al. Nurses' perceptions and practices toward clinical alarms in a transplant cardiac intensive care unit: Exploring key issues leading to alarm fatigue. JMIR Human Factors. 2015;**2**(1):e3

[82] Graham KC, Cvach M. Monitor alarm fatigue: Standardizing use of physiological monitors and decreasing nuisance alarms. American Journal of Critical Care. 2010;**19**(1):28-34

[83] Sendelbach S, Funk M. Alarm fatigue: A patient safety concern. AACN Advanced Critical Care. 2013;**24**(4):378-386

[84] Heine MF, Lake CL. Nature and prevention of errors in anesthesiology. Journal of Surgical Oncology. 2004;**88**(3):143-152

[85] Stawicki SP et al. Natural history of retained surgical items supports the need for team training, early recognition, and prompt retrieval. The American Journal of Surgery. 2014; **208**(1):65-72

[86] Eichhorn JH et al. Standards for patient monitoring during anesthesia at Harvard Medical School. JAMA. 1986;**256**(8):1017-1020

[87] Barlow J, Bayer S, Curry R. Implementing complex innovations in fluid multi-stakeholder environments: Experiences of 'telecare'. Technovation. 2006;**26**(3):396-406

[88] Gander P et al. Fatigue risk management: Organizational factors at the regulatory and industry/company level. Accident Analysis & Prevention. 2011;**43**(2):573-590

[89] Smith A. Franken-algorithms: The Deadly Consequences of Unpredictable Code. 2018. Available from: https://www.theguardian.com/technology/2018/aug/29/coding-algorithms-frankenalgos-program-danger

[90] McGrath SP et al. Surveillance monitoring management for general care units: Strategy, design, and implementation. The Joint Commission Journal on Quality and Patient Safety. 2016;**42**(7):293-302

[91] Taenzer AH, Pyke JB, McGrath SP. A review of current and emerging approaches to address failure-to-rescue. Anesthesiology: The Journal of the American Society of Anesthesiologists. 2011;**115**(2):421-431

[92] Halang W, Colnaric M, Verber D. Supporting high integrity and behavioural predictability of hard real-time systems. Informatica, Special Issue on Parallel and Distributed Real-Time Systems. 1995;**19**:59-69

[93] Du P et al. Soft error resilient QR factorization for hybrid system with GPGPU. Journal of Computational Science. 2013;**4**(6):457-464

[94] Ferek-Petric B. GUI Coding for Identification of Displayable Data Quality from Medical Devices. Google Patents; 2003

[95] Sloan MK, Fennell MJ. Error Detection in Critical Repeating Data in a Wireless Sensor System. Google Patents; 2016

[96] Sukuvaara T et al. A knowledge-based alarm system for monitoring cardiac operated patients—Technical construction and evaluation. International Journal of Clinical Monitoring and Computing. 1993;**10**(2):117-126

[97] Baxt WG, Skora J. Prospective validation of artificial neural network trained to identify acute myocardial infarction. Lancet. 1996;**347**(8993):12-15

[98] Goldman JM, Cordova MJ. Advanced clinical monitoring: Considerations for real-time hemodynamic diagnostics. In: Proceedings of the Annual Symposium on Computer Applications in Medical Care. 1994. pp. 752-756

[99] Laursen P. Event detection on patient monitoring data using causal probabilistic networks. Methods of Information in Medicine. 1994;**33**(1):111-115

Chapter 7

Dangers of Peripheral Intravenous Catheterization: The Forgotten Tourniquet and Other Patient Safety Considerations

Parampreet Kaur, Claire Rickard,
Gregory S. Domer and Kevin R. Glover

Additional information is available at the end of the chapter

http://dx.doi.org/10.5772/intechopen.83854

Abstract

Intravenous catheterization is a widely used invasive procedure, with applications in both ambulatory and hospital settings. Due to its inherently invasive nature, intravenous (IV) therapy is associated with a number of potential complications, many of which are directly relevant to patient safety (PS). PIV-related morbidity may be due to mechanical or nonmechanical factors. The most frequent nonmechanical peripheral venous catheterization adverse events (PVCAEs) include insertion site pain, phlebitis, hematoma formation, and infusate extravasation. The most common mechanical PVCAE is catheter obstruction/occlusion and dislodgement. Significant complications can also occur with the administration of incorrect type or wrong amount of IV fluids. Moreover, simultaneous infusion of incompatible medications can result in infusate precipitation. Finally, less frequent but significant complications have been reported, including bloodstream and local infections, air embolization, nerve damage, arterial puncture, skin necrosis associated with vasopressor infusions, and limb-threatening forgotten tourniquet events. Taken together, the above complications can lead to substantial patient discomfort, unnecessary or prolonged hospitalization, increased costs, and additional downstream morbidity. Efforts to prevent PVCAEs and improve patient outcomes should involve thorough provider education, clinical vigilance by all involved healthcare providers, health service level strategies, as well as the proactive participation of all stakeholders, including patients and their families.

Keywords: complications, intravenous therapy, peripheral intravenous catheter, patient safety

1. Introduction

Intravenous therapy (IVT) is a treatment modality based on infusing various compatible fluids (e.g., solutions, medications, blood, or blood products) directly into a vein [1–3]. Modern clinical efforts at IVT began in the early seventeenth century, but due to complications and generally poor results, the practice was largely abandoned until the nineteenth-century cholera epidemic [4, 5]. Early publications on IVT date back to the 1880s, when Dr. Thomas Latta described its use during the cholera epidemic in Britain [4, 6]. The standard IV use of saline solutions did not begin until the early 1900s. Further advances in IVT occurred in the 1930s, but this modality was not widely available until the 1950s [3, 7, 8]. It was not until the twentieth century, after the two world wars, and the discovery of blood group types and pyrogens, that clinical use of IVT gained more traction [5, 9]. The introduction of plastic bags and IV catheters in the late twentieth century, combined with modern infection control practices, resulted in IVT becoming a widespread and lifesaving therapeutic option [5, 10]. Intravenous administration of fluids in the emergency setting (e.g., trauma, sepsis) can be a lifesaving maneuver and represents the primary method of ensuring adequate intravascular fluid status for patients who are unable to tolerate enteral nutrition [11, 12]. It is estimated that hundreds of millions of PIV catheterizations are performed worldwide each year [13]. The vast majority of these procedures are conducted by nursing staff, with the remainder performed by specialty teams [14]. Of note, approximately 80% of all hospitalized patients receive IVT [15, 16]. At the same time, the frequency of "idle catheters" (e.g., with no active medication or fluid infusion) can be as high as 16%, with approximately 12% reporting at least one sign/symptom of phlebitis [14]. The results of a more recent retrospective cohort study of 3829 patients by Limm et al. showed that 50% of PIVCs inserted in the ED went unused. Of the 43% of patients with idle catheters then admitted to the hospital wards, these continued to be unused 72 h later [17]. There is an increasing awareness (and concern) of the possible morbidity, including life and limb injury, associated with the highly prevalent usage of IVT [18]. The purpose of this chapter is to provide a comprehensive overview of all major complications and patient safety considerations associated with PIVs and IVT in the adult population. In addition, we provide an illustrative case of a "forgotten tourniquet" to illustrate the importance of patient safety measures in this important area of clinical care.

2. Types of venous access

Safe, dependable venous access for infusions is a critical part of patient care. There are two primary types—peripheral and central venous access. The type of access is selected based on the anticipated duration of IVT, the type of medication or solution to be infused, and patient-specific considerations [19, 20]. The focus of this chapter, the PIV catheter, is a short intravenous catheter placed via venipuncture into a peripheral vein, while central venous catheters are inserted into large veins of the central circulation system (e.g., subclavian, jugular, and femoral). Performed an estimated 150–200 million times annually in North America alone, the impact of PIVs is difficult to comprehend [21]. Moreover, up to 8–23% of patients in the emergency department experience difficult PIV placement (e.g., multiple attempts, infiltration, and other placement-related complications). These patients are more likely to require central venous access, which includes significantly higher associated morbidity. Ultrasound-guided PIV catheterization can reduce the need for central venous access, thus potentially reducing morbidity [21]. Not only does the ultrasound-guided PIV access decrease the reliance on central venous access, but it also decreases the overall time, number of attempts, and needle redirections compared to more traditional placement methods [22, 23]. While PIVs are the preferred access mode for short-term IVT, central venous access is utilized for long-term administration of medications or parenteral nutrition [23–27]. At times, when PIV access cannot be established or is quantitatively insufficient for the delivery of desired volume or fluid type, central venous access may be the only viable option to consider [15, 28].

3. Indications and common anatomic sites of peripheral intravenous catheterization

PIV catheterization is indicated for short-term use across a broad range of clinical scenarios, including administration of IV fluids, drugs, blood/blood products, dyes, and contrast media [28, 29]. Several factors must be considered when selecting a site for PIV catheterization. Although common sites of insertion are generally described as the lower arm and the dorsum of the hand, superficial veins of the lower limbs can also be used for cannulation in certain clinical situations [30]. The direct and indirect risks of complications can be curtailed by a more thorough assessment of the vascular anatomy prior to choosing the optimal site, based on both infusion- and patient-related factors [31–35]. Carr et al. reported that the antecubital fossa (ACF), the most common insertion site cannulated in their study of 252 ED patients, was associated with the best rates of insertion success (54.78%), but a secondary analysis revealed that these successfully inserted PIVCs repeatedly failed to last for the intended 3-day dwell time after transfer from the ED to the general hospital units [31]. In a project to reduce infusion pump alarms, Matocha [34] reported that occlusion alarms (60%) represented the highest volume of alarms in a medical oncology unit. After intervention, occlusion alarms were reduced by 17% but still represented the highest volume of alarms, which the author hypothesized might be associated with the majority of catheter placements in the antecubital area due to flexion at the site. Decreasing antecubital area placement in the first place through staff education regarding vascular access planning and insertion competency was suggested as one way of reducing occlusion alarms. Alarm frequency may interfere with patients' sleep, cause unnecessary anxiety, and potentially negatively impact healing [32, 33]. It is imperative to consider the clinical status of the patient carefully before selecting the site. Such assessment should consider the general condition of the veins, tortuosity, locations of valves, bifurcations [36], the size of cannula, type of drug to be administered, infusion rate, and duration of the intended IVT [30]. Intravenous cannula gauge and site of placement are critical factors in defining the success and longevity of PIV cannula [37]. Of note, larger gauge ($P = 0.0002$, RR = 1.17, 95% CI 1.08–1.27) and forearm placement ($P = 0.005$, RR = 0.7, 95% CI 0.55–0.9) are among the strongest predictors of longer functional cannula life [38]. Evidence demonstrates the usefulness of multimodality methodology in improving in first-time insertion success rate [2, 37].

Overall, success rates for PIV placement range between 61 and 90%, with successful insertions being associated with visible or palpable veins, providers with greater procedural volumes, and inserters who were able to predict that placement would be successful [39]. Level of successful venous access also appears to be associated with various patient factors (e.g., age, body mass index, etc.) [40]. Difficult venous access is characterized by non-visible and non-palpable veins for various reasons, including chronic disease, history of intravenous drug use, history of chemotherapy, obesity, or malnourishment [41]. In addition to excellent technical skill and clinical knowledge, various vein visualization devices and ultrasound-based approaches can be helpful in facilitating successful PIV insertion [36]. Such devices include infrared vein visualizers and ultrasound; however, operator experience is required for optimal outcomes and success rates [42]. The ability to leverage adjunctive devices to identify more veins can lead to greater placement and successful and speedier cannulations [40]. In addition, assistive devices may help reduce the number of insertion attempts and diminish complications such as unintended arterial puncture [43, 44].

4. Clinical vignette

A 49-year-old female with type 2 diabetes mellitus and morbid obesity underwent an abdominoplasty due to recurrent lower abdominal cellulitis. Following a series of failed PIV placement attempts in the left forearm, venous access was established on the dorsum of left hand with an 18G cannula. This PIV was then used during the induction of anesthesia, without any apparent problems. The complex operation took approximately 5 h to complete. During this time, fluid replacements were given intravenously. During the procedure, there was no evidence of left upper extremity swelling, color, or temperature change. The point of insertion of the PIV cannula appeared unremarkable when the patient arrived in the postanesthesia care unit (PACU).

Within 4 h, however, the patient reported severe pain in her left hand. This pain persisted despite escalating doses of analgesics. There was a mild but visible swelling in the left hand as compared to the right side, along with decreased capillary refill and distal paresthesia. When the patient's surgeon came to examine the patient, he exposed the entire left upper extremity and discovered an intravenous tourniquet still in place, hiding behind the hospital gown sleeve. The tourniquet was immediately removed, but it was too late to reverse the resultant extremity compartment syndrome. The PIV was also discontinued, and a new catheter is placed in the contralateral hand. An emergency fasciotomy was performed, allowing salvage of the left hand and forearm, at the cost of a large left forearm scar. This substantially increased the length of stay and associated costs and reduced the patient's hospital experience. Fortunately, there were no signs of ischemic injury or permanent nerve damage, and the patient had good functional recovery.

5. Overview of peripheral IV catheter complications

As outlined above, PIV catheters are routinely used for short-term delivery of intravascular fluids and medications, thus being among the most important and the most frequent invasive procedure performed in hospitals. However, PIVs often fail before IVT is completed, with the cited malfunction rate of about 90% [2]. A prospective observational study, the CATHEVAL Project, suggested that the incidence of PVCAEs is significantly underestimated [1]. The incidence rate of at least one PVCAE was 52.3%, with "clinical" PVCAEs occurring significantly more frequently than "mechanical" PVCAEs [1]. The most frequent clinical PVCAEs were phlebitis (20.1/100 PIVs), followed by hematoma (17.7/100 PIVs) and fluid/blood leakage (13.1/100 PIVs). In terms of mechanical complications, obstruction/occlusion of PIV was the most frequent event (12.4/100 PIVs) [1]. Of interest, the authors also reported on post-removal PVCAEs (21.7/100 PIVs) as well as infections (0.4/100 PIVs) [1]. Moreover, significant complications can occur if the incorrect quantity (volume) of IV fluids or incorrect medication infusion/dosage is administered [45, 46].

The prevalence of difficult IV access can be substantial, with one study reporting 23% of patients classified as "moderately difficult" and 5% classified as having "difficult access" [47]. Of interest, female gender and a previous history of several IV placement attempts may be associated with greater risk of difficult venous access, which in turn can increase the overall complication risk [48, 49]. Currently, there is no internationally accepted definition of a "difficult access" patient. Based on clinical observations many have tried to develop a predictive scale to identify adult patients with difficult intravenous access: the DIVA scale [50]. Such scales can be used to recognize patients with high probability of a difficult intravenous access. In such cases various assessment devices (near-infrared and ultrasound) or call for assistance of more experienced individuals in an earlier time frame can prove beneficial to the patient [41, 50].

Globally speaking, prevention of PVCAEs should be the preferred approach, and despite ongoing efforts to improve the current state of affairs, PVCAEs continue to occur, prompting the need for maintaining awareness and reinforcing provider education in this critical important area [18]. In a multicenter prospective study of 1498 patients by Cicolini et al. [51], the authors cited that anatomical site selection and a lack of adherence to in situ PIVC placement recommended guidelines resulted in increased rates of phlebitis. They concluded that additional staff education was needed [51]. DeVries et al. reported a 19% reduction in PIVC-associated bloodstream infections after implementing a fundamental PIVC insertion and education bundle for bedside nurses that increased staff awareness of proper skin preparation, aseptic technique, and the importance of the care and maintenance of dressings [52]. Nursing education leaders in another tertiary healthcare setting developed an educational intervention to improve the recognition and reporting of infiltration and phlebitis on medical-surgical units, which was identified by the risk management database as a concern. Although the differences between pre- and post-knowledge scores were not significant ($P = 0.21$), the unexpected results of the research served as a catalyst to develop annual PIVC procedural education to validate competency related to PIVC-related complications [53].

A standardized approach to education and competency assessment across the healthcare system is recommended. A simulation-based multimodal educational method should be considered, including self-study and deliberate practice, with objective outcome monitoring and feedback using well-designed, validated, and reliable checklists [36, 54–56]. After all, it is the responsibility of the entire healthcare team to monitor for signs and symptoms of PVCAEs and intervene in a timely and appropriate fashion [30].

Subsequent paragraphs of this chapter will discuss PVCAEs grouped into "localized" or "systemic" categories.

6. Local PVCAEs

Phlebitis: Phlebitis is an inflammation of the vein and causes pain, swelling, redness, and tenderness. It can be caused by various sources like mechanical, chemical, or infective insults to the vein [2]. The mechanical cause; irritation with cannula rubbing the vein, chemical cause; medications with a hypertonic or acidic/alkaline solution, or an infective phlebitis; microorganism entering the vein through the puncture site can cause the inflammation [30]. *Diagnosis:* It is one of the most talked about complication in the literature [2]. The diagnosis of superficial phlebitis can be made by physical examination of the site. Redness, warmth, tenderness, and swelling along the course of the vein can help make the diagnosis, although there are more than 70 tools used in the literature and none well validated [57]. In certain cases, an ultrasound of the affected area is needed to make or ignore the diagnosis. *Prevention and treatment*: Most complications are preventable if simple hand hygiene and safe principles are observed at every point of contact with the patient [2]. According to a recent secondary analysis, the antecubital fossa is associated with lower phlebitis rates as compared with upper arm and wrist veins [37]. Another systemic review showed that the antecubital veins had lower rate of phlebitis as compared to hand veins [58]. The treatment of phlebitis depends on the location, extent, symptom, and underlying medical conditions. Typically, it should be removed and documented with the time, date, and reason of removal [59]. Documentation can improve the staff compliance and help to improve quality of care of the patients with PIVC [60, 61]. Superficial phlebitis can be treated by applying warm compresses, elevation of the involved extremity, and oral or topical anti-inflammatory medications. External compression with fitted stockings may be beneficial for lower extremity superficial phlebitis. If left untreated, superficial phlebitis can complicate to local infection and abscess formation, clot formation, and progression to a deep venous thrombosis and pulmonary embolism. Deep vein thrombosis can further lead to postphlebitic syndrome.

Tissue infiltration and extravasation: Tissue infiltration occurs when the infusate solution is inadvertently administered (or leaks out) into the surrounding tissues. It can be caused by improper placement, dislodgement, or distal puncture/erosion of the catheter and can be associated with relative movement of the patient and the catheter. Extravasation arises when a solution or medication is administered and inadvertently leaks into the surrounding tissues, causing tissue damage. This unintended leakage can be caused by the same reasons as infiltration, including improper placement or dislodgement of the catheter. Certain sites are more prone to extravasation injuries like dorsum of the foot, ankle, antecubital fossa, and the areas near joints where there is little protection for underlying structures [18]. Of interest, extravasations tend to be more common during night hours and thus may be more likely to go undetected, even in closely monitored situations. Extravasation is more likely to occur in patients with fragile, mobile, thrombosed, and difficult to cannulate veins [18]. The degree of subsequent cellular injury is determined by the volume of the infiltrating solution and physiochemical characteristics, such as pH, osmolarity, and dissociability [18]. *Diagnosis*: The diagnosis of infiltration is usually made by observing local tissue edema, cool skin with blanching, and decreased (or stopped) flow rate. The patient usually complains of discomfort, burning, and tightness of the involved extremity/ anatomic location [62]. Comparison to the contralateral limb may help confirm this diagnosis. In the case of extravasation, signs and symptoms may be similar to infiltration but will additionally include burning, irritation, redness, blistering, mottling, ulceration, or permanent damage like necrosis of the affected tissue. The damage can spread to involve nerves, tendons, and joints even months after the original insult [18]. It can additionally include disfigurement, complex regional pain syndrome, and loss of function [63]. *Prevention and treatment:* Prevention of infiltration includes the avoidance of PIV placement in the hand, antecubital fossa, and upper arm, properly securing the catheter and monitoring the IV site frequently [2, 36]. It is important to check the patient's pulse and capillary refill [64]. Clinical management includes stopping the infusion, removing the PIV, elevating the limb, and general measures to alleviate patient discomfort. It has also been reported that local application of hyaluronidase may help, primarily through breaking down subcutaneous cellular components and speeding up the reabsorption of the extravasated fluids [65, 66]. Finally, the original infusion should be restarted at a different site, with all pertinent interventions documented in the medical record.

Prevention of extravasation includes careful placement of PIV cannula, close monitoring of active intravenous fluid infusions, flushing the catheter with sterile saline to ensure patency, and the use of suitable dressings and securements to prevent undue movement [18]. Once extravasation is recognized, the infusion needs to be stopped and the cannula removed. This is especially important when the medication/fluid being infused is potentially toxic to local tissues. Palpable effusion in the subcutaneous tissues may need to be drained, and the limb should be immobilized and elevated above the level of the heart. Application of cold packs can provide symptomatic relief. Indications for surgery include full-thickness skin necrosis, ulceration, and persistent pain [67]. If appropriate treatment is delayed, surgical debridement, skin grafting, and amputation may be the end result of such an injury [18].

Hemorrhage/hematoma: Hemorrhage is defined as bleeding from the puncture site, while hematoma is a localized collection of extravasated blood, usually clotted, within an organ or tissue. Both hemorrhage and hematoma may be caused by blood leaking out of the vein into the tissue due to puncture or trauma. The COSMOS study found that PIV catheters based on a compact closed system were associated with lower rate of hematomas when compared to a mounted open system [68]. Patients who receive antiplatelet therapy or therapeutic anticoagulation are especially predisposed to hematoma/ecchymosis formation [69]. *Diagnosis*: The signs and symptoms of swelling, tenderness, and reddish discoloration at the site are usually sufficient to diagnose PIV-related hematoma. *Prevention and treatment*: The first management step is the application of appropriate localized pressure until the bleeding stops. This is followed by a sterile transparent dressing that can prevent hematoma formation or expansion. Proper PIV insertion, frequent monitoring of the site, and application of pressure after removal of cannula can help prevent hemorrhage and formation of hematoma. At the same time, patients, providers, and nurses should be mindful of using extended external compression times at the insertion site, especially in older patients with impaired skin conditions, as this can lead to further tissue injury [1]. The majority of PIV-related bleeding and hematomas are fortunately self-limited.

Nerve injury: When tissue infiltration associated with a PIV catheter affects a nerve coursing the surrounding tissues, nerve injury can occur. It is also possible for the IV needle to lacerate, puncture, and potentially injure a nerve. Finally, localized bleeding/hematoma may irritate a nerve. *Diagnosis*: Patients may not experience any discomfort in the beginning, but it is possible for localized numbness or tingling, loss of sensation to pin prick to emerge later on [70, 71]. Nerve injury can range from neurapraxia with complete recovery (minor injury) to neurotmesis with Wallerian degeneration distal to the site of injury (severe injury) [70]. *Prevention and treatment*: The avoidance of nerve injury requires good procedural skills and knowledge of pertinent anatomy. The PIV placing provider should be conscious of venipuncture sites associated with the greatest risk, including the distal sensory branches of the radial and ulnar nerves for sites in the dorsal hand, the superficial radial nerve at the cephalic vein of the radial wrist, the median nerve on the volar aspects of the wrist, the median and anterior interosseous nerves at or above the antecubital fossa, and the lateral and medial antebrachial nerves for the antecubital fossa [36]. The needle insertion should be as shallow as possible, preferably at an angle of 5–15° relative to the skin and using the non-dominant arm [71]. Although nerve injury is rare, the patient should still be aware of this complication and encouraged to inform the nurse immediately if he or she experiences any strange sensation during PIV placement. Nerve damage tends to be self-limited, with typical recovery times of a few weeks or months. Surgical exploration may be required in patients with intractable pain, severe functional loss, or those without recovery signs within 3–6 months after the initial injury [72–74].

Occlusion: Occlusion is defined as the slowing or cessation of fluid infusion. It can occur due to the mechanical blockage within the cannula or fibrin deposition in/around the tip of the cannula. In addition, it may be due to swollen phlebitic veins, or insertion at a point of flexion, both of which may collapse the catheter and prevent flow [75]. There may be a higher incidence of occlusion associated with insertion in the hand, antecubital fossa, or upper arm, when compared to forearm placement [2, 37]. 25.6% had failed catheterization due to PIV occlusions in an analysis from a randomized controlled trial in Australia. The occlusion was associated with infusions of antibiotics, hydrocortisone, in the setting of concurrent infection, and the use of subsequent (rather than initial) catheters [37]. In a single-center prospective study done in Australia, catheter failure due to occlusion/infiltration was reported to be 14%. In the same study, flucloxacillin, female gender, and 22-gauge PIVs were significant predictors of occlusion [49]. *Diagnosis*: Occlusion can be diagnosed by the presence of discomfort, blood within the line, or PIV not running. *Prevention and treatment*: Actively checking for kinks and removing nonfunctioning cannulas will help reduce the overall duration of functional occlusion. Insertion of PIV by a trained specialist may also help reduce the risk of occlusion [37]. Various methods have been tried to prevent occlusion. In recent randomized trial, the rate of occlusion was lower with heparin infusion compared to placebo infusion [59].

Dislodgement: Dislodgement can occur when IV catheter was incorrectly secured with standard medical tape or another adhesive securement device. More frequently, catheters that are correctly secured become dislocated when more forces are applied upon the catheter than the securement method was intended to endure. IV dislodgement can lead to an unscheduled IV restart or more invasive central line. Dislodgement rate has been reported in the range of 3.7–9.9% in a prospective randomized study with a mean of 6.9%. Even a greater rate of 17.5%

was observed in prospective observational studies [2]. At almost 10% dislodgement rate, financial dislodgement burden can be tremendous translating to 33 million, if approximately 330 million IV catheters are sold in the USA [76]. *Diagnosis:* Cannula location is estimated by the flow of IV fluids and/or IV flushes. To evaluate PIVC fiction or dislodgement, we need to ask questions like does the IV flush easily and does the IV fluid flow easily? *Prevention and treatment*: Transparent and semipermeable polyurethane or sterile gauze and tape dressing are both recommended [77, 78]. Catheters with stabilization features like wings may help to secure the catheter due of an additional adhesive dressing contact area [79]. To decrease catheter movement and increase the adhesive surface area, attaching extension tubing to the catheter hub may prove beneficial [80]. Effective securement reduces the motion within the vessel which can in turn minimize the irritation, inflammation, occlusion, and risk of infection [77, 81]. At the same time, increase in catheter complex bulk may make the catheter more vulnerable to displacement due to clothing grabbing onto the catheter complex [38].

Venous spasm: Venous spasm is a complication of various minor procedures, including PIV insertion and arterial line placement [82]. Venous spasm can occur in the presence of cold IV fluid infusion, drug-related irritation, or trauma to the vein during insertion [82–84]. *Diagnosis:* The signs and symptoms of pain, blanching at the insertion site, slowing of IV infusion, and difficulty in palpating the vein can help facilitate the diagnosis. *Prevention and treatment:* Applying a warm compress, slowing the infusion rate, and potential application of a topical vasodilator, in addition to patient reassurance [82, 85] See **Table 1**.

7. Systemic complications

Air embolism: Air embolism is defined as an unintended venous administration of air through an intravenous access device or insertion site. It is usually associated with central venous catheters but can also occur with peripheral intravenous central catheters and less commonly with short peripheral catheters. The incidence of this complication may be low, but it is potentially fatal, with reported mortality as high as 30% [86]. Clinical signs and symptoms may vary depending on the patient, rate of infusion, volume of air, and anatomical location [87]. Physiologic injury can be due to associated ischemia, infarction, thrombotic, or inflammatory response. *Diagnosis:* Clinical signs and symptoms of air embolism may be nonspecific and not readily recognizable, yet immediate intervention is critical to adequately address the problem and prevent/minimize associated harm. Patient may present with sudden onset of dyspnea, cough, wheezing, chest or shoulder pain, tachypnea, tachycardia, hypotension, and/or neurological findings of cerebrovascular accidents [86, 88]. *Prevention and treatment*: For peripherally inserted catheters, prevention includes the avoidance of air, both primarily and by so-called "air traps" built into the IV circuit. When placing and removing central venous catheters, the patient should be placed in Trendelenburg (during catheter removal), followed by supine (subsequent 20–30 min) position. Prompt diagnosis and focused treatment are mandatory in cases of air embolism. After stabilizing the patient, immediate evaluation and management should be instituted [89]. Affected patients should be transferred to intensive care for close monitoring, with considerations given to hyperbaric oxygen therapy as an adjunct [88].

Pulmonary edema: Pulmonary edema or fluid overload is caused by excess fluid accumulation in the lungs, due to excessive fluid in the circulatory system [90]. Elderly, pregnant women, children, infants, and patients with cardiac, pulmonary, or renal disease are at risk of developing hypervolemia. In the context of IVT, fluid overload usually represents a combination of errors, from miscalculated IV rate, to inadvertently prolonged infusion, to lack of diagnostic recognition of early clinical symptoms. *Diagnosis:* Patients usually present with restlessness, breathlessness, tachycardia, dyspnea, cyanosis, and pink frothy sputum. Chest radiography can show typical findings of cephalization, interstitial edema, pulmonary vein enlargement, hilar fullness, Kerley lines, cardiomegaly, and pleural effusion [91]. Associated findings may include decreased oxygen saturation, increased respiratory rate, and pulmonary crackles on auscultation. Finally, increased body weight (e.g., "water weight") may be noted [92]. *Prevention and treatment*: The diagnosis of acute fluid overload requires immediate medical attention and treatment. This involves stopping the infusion, raising the head of the bed, applying oxygen, taking vital signs, complete cardiovascular assessment, diuresis when indicated, and appropriate education of the involved medical providers.

Catheter fragment embolism: Intravascular embolization of catheter fragment is a rare complication that occurs when a small part of the cannula breaks off and flows into the vascular system [93, 94]. *Diagnosis:* Symptomatology and diagnostic identification of intravascular embolization of catheter fragments are variable, largely depending on the location and size of the object. Most events are completely asymptomatic and only found incidentally on imaging performed for unrelated reasons [94]. Larger fragments, especially those that migrate into more central venous and pulmonary circulation, may result in palpitations, arrhythmias, chest pain, shortness of breath, cough, pain, and/or hypotension [86]. Chest X-rays may help assess the presence of any fragment. *Prevention and treatment*: Prevention starts with a careful inspection of the cannula and more specifically its distal end, to see if the PIV is structurally intact. Catheters should not be removed against unexpected resistance, which should prompt further investigation (e.g., ultrasound) before proceeding. PIV devices should be protected from twisting, bending, entanglement, etc. Repairs should only be done through official channels involving the manufacturer. Each event should be documented and disclosed to patients and their families, in accordance with existing guidelines [86].

Infection: Local infection is caused by lack of asepsis at insertion or regrowth of skin bacteria which then enter the PIV site. It can present as purulent drainage from the site; usually after 2–3 days it takes the body to mount a response after PIV placement. The majority of serious bloodstream infections are associated with central venous catheters, especially when catheters are placed emergently or used for prolonged periods of time [59]. For PIV catheters, the situation is different, since these are placed in less acutely unwell patients and typically require shorter periods of hospitalization and IVT. Although bacterial colonization of PIV catheters can increase with dwelling times of more than 72 h, there does not seem to be an elevated risk of associated phlebitis or infection regardless of whether the PIC catheter is replaced due to clinical indication or subject to routine replacement between 72 and 96 h [1, 2, 95, 96]. Thus, international guidelines now recommend removal of PIVCs when treatment is completed or sooner if any complication develops [97, 98]. Despite the

http://dx.doi.org/10.5772/intechopen.83854

Peripheral venous catheter adverse events (PVCAEs)	
Local complications	**Systemic complications**
Tissue infiltration and extravasation Infusate solution leaks out into the surrounding tissue *Diagnosis*: detecting local tissue edema, cool skin, decreased flow rate, and comparison with contralateral limb *Prevention:* avoiding PIV too close to the joint, securing the catheter, and monitoring site frequently	**Air embolism** Rare unintended venous administration of air through IV site *Diagnosis:* nonspecific sudden onset of dyspnea, cough, wheezing, tachypnea, and/or neurological signs of CVAs *Prevention:* avoidance of air-traps in IV circuit; patient is in Trendelenburg position followed by supine position during catheter removal
Hemorrhage/hematoma Bleeding from puncture site/localized collection of extravasated blood *Diagnosis*: swelling, tenderness, and reddish discoloration *Prevention:* application of pressure after removal of cannula, usage of sterile transparent dressing	**Pulmonary edema** Fluid overload caused by excess fluid accumulation in the lungs *Diagnosis:* breathlessness, tachycardia, dyspnea, cyanosis, pink frothy sputum, chest radiography, decreased oxygen saturation *Prevention:* avoidance of miscalculation IV rate and prolonged infusion, early recognition of symptoms
Nerve injury Due to tissue infiltration, IV needle laceration, hematoma irritation *Diagnosis:* localized numbness or tingling, loss of sensation to pin prick *Prevention:* good knowledge of anatomy, shallow insertion at 5–15 degrees relative to the skin	**Catheter fragment embolism** Small part of the cannula breaks off and flows into the vascular system *Diagnosis:* symptomatology depends on the location, incidental finding on imaging, chest X-ray *Prevention:* careful inspection of cannula; catheters should not be removed against unexpected resistance; repairs should only be done by manufacturer
Occlusion Slowing or cessation of fluid infusion *Diagnosis:* presence of discomfort, blood within the PV line, PIV not running *Prevention:* check the kinks; remove the nonfunctioning cannula	**Infection** Purulent discharge from the site after 2–3 days *Diagnosis:* presence of purulent discharge, and/or temperature, blood count, D-dimer *Prevention:* hand hygiene, aseptic technique
Dislodgement Due to more forces applied upon the catheter than the securement method was intended to endure *Diagnosis:* checking the flow of IV fluids or IV flushes *Prevention:* effective securement; use of catheters with wings, extension tubing for movement	**Hypersensitivity** A severe hypersensitivity can be life- threatening *Diagnosis:* sudden fever, joint swelling, rash, urticarial, bronchospasm, wheezing *Prevention:* ask about any previous history of allergies, stay with the patient for five to ten minutes to detect early signs
Venous spasm Due to cold IV fluid infusion, drug-related irritation, or trauma to the vein *Diagnosis:* pain, blanching at the site, difficulty in palpating vein *Prevention:* apply warm compress; slow infusion rate	**Intra-arterial placement** Misplacement of PIV due to lack of vigilance *Diagnosis:* detection of pulsatile blood, changes in capillary refill, appearance of ischemia, blood gas analysis, ultrasound *Prevention:* recollecting that veins are more superficial than arteries, immediate removal of PIV after detecting pulsatile bleeding

Table 1. Local and systemic complications of peripheral venous catheter.

low occurrence of both local and bloodstream infections involving PIV catheters, severe infections can still significantly contribute to patient morbidity simply because of the ubiquitous nature of peripheral catheters [59]. *Diagnosis:* Local infection can be diagnosed by signs and symptoms of tenderness, swelling, erythema, purulent drainage, temperature, and appropriate laboratory testing (e.g., comprehensive blood count or D-dimer in cases of phlebitis) [99]. Of note, lower extremity PIVs are associated with higher incidence of infections when compared to upper extremity PIVs [100]. *Prevention and treatment*: To reduce morbidity and financial burden of PIV-related infections, appropriate education and multidisciplinary efforts should be implemented. For all PIV catheters, a clean, dry, intact dressing is recommended because any soilage will facilitate microorganism growth. Any soilage covered by nontransparent dressings can increase the risk of not detecting infection [1]. The density of skin flora at the site plays an important role in infection. From purely procedural perspective, the first and essential parts of the process should involve removal of the infected PIV cannula and cleansing of the site using sterile technique. Hand hygiene, clipping of excess hair, skin preparation with alcoholic chlorhexidine solution, proper aseptic technique, and maximal sterile barriers including cap, mask, sterile gown, and gloves during insertion can reduce the incidence of infection [59]. During the PIV insertion process, the antiseptic scrubbing technique also modulates the risk of infection [76]. Post-insertion, infection prevention is still crucial and is achieved by meticulous attention to hand hygiene, aseptic preparation of injectates and infusates, needleless connector decontamination with effective antiseptic, and technique. The insertion site requires weekly redressing (or sooner if the dressing is compromised), including recleaning of the insertion site with alcoholic chlorhexidine. Under certain circumstances, such as neutropenic patients, filling and flushing the lumen of the catheter with an antibiotic solution may provide some prophylactic benefits [59]. A final and very simple way to prevent PIVC-associated infections is to ensure the PIVC is reviewed daily and documented, and there is consideration of removal, for example, with the patient moved to oral medication [101] and vigilance for "idle PIVCs" See **Table 1**.

8. Special topics

Intra-arterial placement and injection: An intra-arterial misplacement of PIV, including the initiation of intra-arterial infusion, occurs seldom but is considered a matter of serious concern. Although the precise number of inadvertent intra-arterial PIV cannulation and subsequent injection is unknown, the frequency has been estimated to be as low as 1 in 56,000 and as high as 1 in 3440 [102]. However, the potential consequences of missing the diagnosis can be devastating. If not promptly recognized, its consequences may include arterial spasm, distal ischemia, and eventual development of limb-threatening gangrene [103]. Risk factors associated with unintentional arterial PIV placement include morbid obesity, dark skin, lack of patient cooperation, significant hypotension, and lack of vigilance [103, 104]. *Diagnosis:* Diagnosis can be made by detecting red pulsatile blood, observing changes in capillary refill, the presence of intense pain, and/or the appearance of distal ischemia. Confirmation is done by blood gas analysis, pressure transducer placement, and ultrasound [104]. *Prevention and treatment*: Prevention is the most important measure in this setting. Providers must take great care that the PIV catheter is inserted into a vein, remembering that peripheral veins tend to be more superficial than arteries. Except for very few clinical circumstances (e.g., catastrophic hypotension), arterial cannulation will result in readily visible, pulsatile bleeding from the PIV catheter. In the case of inadvertent intra-arterial injection, it is primarily the intravenous drug that will be most likely to contribute to subsequent problems, as opposed to the ordinary intravenous electrolyte solution. Management consists of PIV catheter removal, assurance of hemostasis, prevention/management of vasospasm, and treatment of any distal complications See **Table 1**.

Forgotten tourniquet: Phlebotomy tourniquets are simple devices used to temporarily restrict venous blood flow, making veins more prominent and easier to see prior to PIV catheter placement. Some considerations regarding the use of tourniquets include the need for optimized location of placement (3–4 inches above intended PIV site), avoiding too much tension to prevent tourniquet from rolling up on itself/twisting and causing discomfort and releasing the tension within approximately 1 min of application [105]. Fortunately a rare occurrence, a phlebotomy tourniquet left in place for prolonged periods of time (e.g., hours) can result in the development of extremity compartment syndrome—a potentially limb-threatening condition [106, 107]. Compartment syndrome is a serious injury defined by an increase in pressure within a fascia-enclosed muscle compartment that results in compromised circulation leading to nerve damage and muscle necrosis [108]. This can lead to permanent disability, amputation, or even death from the release of toxic metabolites. Many of the above findings may not be present until late in the disease process. Thus, early diagnosis is imperative [109, 110]. A high degree of suspicion is crucial to allow an early diagnosis. Pain requiring analgesia in the extremity with the PIV should raise awareness and prompt a thorough examination of the entire extremity. Diagnosis can be especially challenging in children, intubated and sedated patients, and patients with neurological compromise or altered mental status. Increased vigilance must occur in these patients. If compartment syndrome is suspected once a "forgotten tourniquet" event occurs, an urgent surgical consult should be obtained. To prevent this serious omission and thus improve PS, appropriate education/training and procedural checklist implementation may be helpful [111]. Such occurrences, due to the potential for associated patient harm, should be viewed and treated as sentinel events [112]. In addition to compartment syndrome, this complication can also lead to the development of deep vein thrombosis in the affected limb [107]. This chapter's *Clinical Vignette* was based on a hypothetical scenario involving this rare but potentially severe occurrence.

9. Discussion

Due to its ubiquitous nature, IVT is associated with significant number of complications, both in terms of absolute quantity and taxonomy. In a recent survey, approximately one-third of pediatric patients and one-fourth of adult patients reported experiences involving a potentially preventable IVT-related complication. As outlined throughout this book series, patient safety is a "team sport" [111, 112]. Consequently, active participation of all stakeholders is required to optimize patient outcomes. This involves active involvement of all those who directly or indirectly participate in IVT—providers, patients, and families. Our *Clinical Vignette* demonstrates the dangers inherently associated with increasingly complex systems, where transitions of care occur frequently and where several different teams care for the same patient over a period of just several hours. In such environments, even the smallest mistake can result in catastrophic sequelae.

In this chapter, we outlined key considerations around two primary types of PVCAEs—local and systemic. We also discussed intra-arterial PIV catheter placement and the rare but devastating scenario involving the "forgotten tourniquet." Each topic was presented in a clinically relevant fashion, incorporating a brief description, diagnosis, management, and finally prevention. Clinical approach to preventing PVCAEs is multipronged and includes a broad variety of considerations, such as checklists, knowledge of procedures and equipment, proper sterile technique, and the maintenance of appropriate PIV site cleanliness. Providers must also be aware of subtle clinical signs of PVCAEs, including PIV site erythema, IVT-related tissue injury, manifestations of air embolization, and signs of PIV catheter occlusion [2, 113]. In addition, each of the sections outlined specific strategies to prevent PVCAEs and PIV catheter failure. With growing numbers of patients needing vascular access for a range IVTs, providers need to show an understanding of the broad range of vascular access devices and corresponding clinical management aspects, including specific indications for various device types. Finally, providers need to be aware of patient needs, preferences, and concerns. After all, for many patients it is not the procedure that is of maximum concern but rather the clinician's communication skills, competence, and appropriate selection of PIV insertion site [114]. Patients and their families may be greatly untapped allies in preventing, monitoring, and reporting adverse events [101].

10. Conclusion

In summary, PVCAEs continue to be quite common and can lead to substantial patient discomfort, unnecessary or prolonged hospitalization, increased costs, and additional downstream morbidity. To improve patient outcomes, enhance patient safety, and reduce healthcare costs, there has been a substantial interest to implement measures aimed at reducing the incidence of PVCAEs [2]. Efforts to prevent PVCAEs should involve thorough provider education, clinical vigilance by all involved healthcare providers, as well as the proactive participation of all stakeholders, including patients and their families.

Acknowledgements

The authors would like to thank Dr. Stanislaw P. Stawicki for providing generous assistance and input regarding this chapter and its scientific content.

Author details

Parampreet Kaur[1]*, Claire Rickard[2,3,4], Gregory S. Domer[5] and Kevin R. Glover[6]

*Address all correspondence to: parampreet.kaur@sluhn.org

1 Department of Research and Innovation, St. Luke's University Health Network, Bethlehem, Pennsylvania, United States

2 National Centre of Research Excellence in Nursing Interventions, Alliance for Vascular Access Teaching and Research (AVATAR), Menzies Health Institute Queensland, Griffith University, Australia

3 Centre for Clinical Nursing, Royal Brisbane and Women's Hospital, Australia

4 Princess Alexandra Hospital, Woolloongabba, Australia

5 Department of Surgery, Division of Vascular Surgery, St. Luke's University Health Network, Bethlehem, Pennsylvania, United States

6 B. Braun Medical, Inc., Bethlehem, Pennsylvania, USA

References

[1] Miliani K et al. Peripheral venous catheter-related adverse events: Evaluation from a multicentre epidemiological study in France (the CATHEVAL Project). PLoS One. 2017;**12**(1):e0168637

[2] Helm RE et al. Accepted but unacceptable: Peripheral IV catheter failure. Journal of Infusion Nursing. 2015;**38**(3):189-203

[3] Plumer AL. Plumer's Principles and Practice of Intravenous Therapy. Philadelphia, PA: Lippincott Williams & Wilkins; 2007

[4] Cosnett JE. The origins of intravenous fluid therapy. The Lancet. 1989;**333**(8641):768-771

[5] Barsoum N, Kleeman C. Now and then, the history of parenteral fluid administration. American Journal of Nephrology. 2002;**22**(2-3):284-289

[6] Foëx BA. How the cholera epidemic of 1831 resulted in a new technique for fluid resuscitation. Emergency Medicine Journal. 2003;**20**(4):316-318

[7] Jenkins M. History of fluid administration during anesthesia and operation. In: Anaesthesia. Switzerland: Springer; 1985. pp. 102-107

[8] Awad S, Allison SP, Lobo DN. The history of 0.9% saline. Clinical Nutrition. 2008; **27**(2):179-188

[9] Millam D. The history of intravenous therapy. Journal of Intravenous Nursing: The Official Publication of the Intravenous Nurses Society. 1996;**19**(1):5-14

[10] Rivera A et al. The history of peripheral intravenous catheters: How little plastic tubes revolutionized medicine. Acta Anaesthesiologica Belgica. 2005;**56**(3):271

[11] Boyd JH et al. Fluid resuscitation in septic shock: A positive fluid balance and elevated central venous pressure are associated with increased mortality. Critical Care Medicine. 2011;**39**(2):259-265

[12] Nolan J, Parr M. Aspects of resuscitation in trauma. British Journal of Anaesthesia. 1997;**79**(2):226-240

[13] Soifer NE et al. Prevention of peripheral venous catheter complications with an intravenous therapy team: A randomized controlled trial. Archives of Internal Medicine. 1998;**158**(5):473-477

[14] Alexandrou E et al. International prevalence of the use of peripheral intravenous catheters. Journal of Hospital Medicine. 2015;**10**(8):530-533

[15] Waitt C, Waitt P, Pirmohamed M. Intravenous therapy. Postgraduate Medical Journal. 2004;**80**(939):1-6

[16] Tjon JA, Ansani NT. Transdermal nitroglycerin for the prevention of intravenous infusion failure due to phlebitis and extravasation. Annals of Pharmacotherapy. 2000;**34**(10):1189-1192

[17] Limm EI et al. Half of all peripheral intravenous lines in an Australian tertiary emergency department are unused: Pain with no gain? Annals of Emergency Medicine. 2013;**62**(5):521-525

[18] Al-Benna S, O'Boyle C, Holley J. Extravasation injuries in adults. ISRN Dermatology. 2013;**2013**:856541

[19] Horattas MC et al. Changing concepts in long-term central venous access: Catheter selection and cost savings. American Journal of Infection Control. 2001;**29**(1):32-40

[20] Cheung E et al. Venous access: A practical review for 2009. Canadian Family Physician. 2009;**55**(5):494-496

[21] Gottlieb M et al. Ultrasound-guided peripheral intravenous line placement: A narrative review of evidence-based best practices. Western Journal of Emergency Medicine. 2017;**18**(6):1047-1054

[22] Doniger SJ et al. Randomized controlled trial of ultrasound-guided peripheral intravenous catheter placement versus traditional techniques in difficult-access pediatric patients. Pediatric Emergency Care. 2009;**25**(3):154-159

[23] Au AK et al. Decrease in central venous catheter placement due to use of ultrasound guidance for peripheral intravenous catheters. The American Journal of Emergency Medicine. 2012;**30**(9):1950-1954

[24] Pittiruti M et al. ESPEN guidelines on parenteral nutrition: Central venous catheters (access, care, diagnosis and therapy of complications). Clinical Nutrition. 2009; **28**(4):365-377

[25] Gallieni M, Pittiruti M, Biffi R. Vascular access in oncology patients. CA: A Cancer Journal for Clinicians. 2008;**58**(6):323-346

[26] Dychter SS et al. Intravenous therapy: A review of complications and economic considerations of peripheral access. Journal of Infusion Nursing. 2012;**35**(2):84-91

[27] Gerlach AT et al. Does delaying early intravenous fat emulsion during parenteral nutrition reduce infections during critical illness? Surgical Infections. 2011;**12**(1):43-47

[28] Lowell JA, Bothe A Jr. Venous access: Preoperative, operative, and postoperative dilemmas. Surgical Clinics of North America. 1991;**71**(6):1231-1246

[29] Nentwich PF. Intravenous Therapy: A Comprehensive Application of Intravenous Therapy and Medication Administration. Boston: Jones & Bartlett Learning; 1990

[30] McCallum L, Higgins D. Care of peripheral venous cannula sites. Nursing Times. 2012; **108**(34-35):12 14-15

[31] Carr PJ et al. Insertion of peripheral intravenous cannulae in the emergency department: Factors associated with first-time insertion success. The Journal of Vascular Access. 2016;**17**(2):182-190

[32] Sowan AK et al. Changes in default alarm settings and standard In-service are insufficient to improve alarm fatigue in an intensive care unit: A pilot project. JMIR Human Factors. 2016;**3**(1):e1

[33] Cvach M. Monitor alarm fatigue: An integrative review. Biomedical Instrumentation & Technology. 2012;**46**(4):268-277

[34] Matocha D. Reducing infusion pump alarms through structured interventions. The Journal of the Association for Vascular Access. 2018;**23**(2):87-95

[35] Carr PJ et al. Development of a clinical prediction rule to improve peripheral intravenous cannulae first attempt success in the emergency department and reduce post insertion failure rates: The Vascular Access Decisions in the Emergency Room (VADER) study protocol. BMJ Open. 2016;**6**(2):e009196

[36] Journal of Infusion Nursing. 2016;**39**(1S):S1-S157. Available from: https://source.yiboshi.com/20170417/1492425631944540325.pdf

[37] Wallis MC et al. Risk factors for peripheral intravenous catheter failure: A multivariate analysis of data from a randomized controlled trial. Infection Control and Hospital Epidemiology. 2014;**35**(1):63-68

[38] Dillon MF et al. Factors that affect longevity of intravenous cannulas: A prospective study. QJM: An International Journal of Medicine. 2008;**101**(9):731-735

[39] Carr PJ et al. Tools, clinical prediction rules, and algorithms for the insertion of peripheral intravenous catheters in adult hospitalized patients: A systematic scoping review of literature. Journal of Hospital Medicine. 2017;**12**(10):851-858

[40] Chiao FB et al. Vein visualization: Patient characteristic factors and efficacy of a new infrared vein finder technology. British Journal of Anaesthesia. 2013;**110**(6):966-971

[41] Sou V et al. A clinical pathway for the management of difficult venous access. BMC Nursing. 2017;**16**(1):64

[42] Rippey JC et al. Predicting and preventing peripheral intravenous cannula insertion failure in the emergency department: Clinician 'gestalt' wins again. Emergency Medicine Australasia. 2016;**28**(6):658-665

[43] Froehlich CD et al. Ultrasound-guided central venous catheter placement decreases complications and decreases placement attempts compared with the landmark technique in patients in a pediatric intensive care unit. Critical Care Medicine. 2009;**37**(3):1090-1096

[44] Vogel JA et al. Is long axis view superior to short axis view in ultrasound-guided central venous catheterization? Critical Care Medicine. 2015;**43**(4):832-839

[45] Ferner RE, Aronson JK. Clarification of terminology in medication errors. Drug Safety. 2006;**29**(11):1011-1022

[46] Mangino MJ et al. Crystalloid and Colloid Resuscitation: Hypertonic Saline, Starches, Polymers, and Gelatins. Hemorrhagic Shock: Recognition, Pathophysiology, and Management. Hauppauge, NY: Nova Publishers; 2017

[47] Witting MD. IV access difficulty: Incidence and delays in an urban emergency department. The Journal of Emergency Medicine. 2012;**42**(4):483-487

[48] Armenteros-Yeguas V et al. Prevalence of difficult venous access and associated risk factors in highly complex hospitalised patients. Journal of Clinical Nursing. 2017; **26**(23-24):4267-4275

[49] Marsh N et al. Observational study of peripheral intravenous catheter outcomes in adult hospitalized patients: A multivariable analysis of peripheral intravenous catheter failure. Journal of Hospital Medicine. 2018;**13**(2):83-89

[50] van Loon FHJ et al. Development of the A-DIVA scale: A clinical predictive scale to identify difficult intravenous access in adult patients based on clinical observations. Medicine. 2016;**95**(16):e3428-e3428

[51] Cicolini G et al. Phlebitis risk varies by peripheral venous catheter site and increases after 96 hours: A large multi-Centre prospective study. Journal of Advanced Nursing. 2014;**70**(11):2539-2549

[52] DeVries M, Valentine M, Mancos P. Protected clinical indication of peripheral intravenous lines: Successful implementation. The Journal of the Association for Vascular Access. 2016;**21**(2):89-92

[53] Woody G, Davis BA. Increasing nurse competence in peripheral intravenous therapy. Journal of Infusion Nursing. 2013;**36**(6):413-419

[54] Study Published in the Journal of the Association for Vascular Access Offers Evidence to Support the Use of B. Braun Medical's Peripheral IV Checklist to Measure Procedural Performance of Clinicians. May 2017, GLOBE NEWSWIRE

[55] Keleekai NL et al. Improving nurses' peripheral intravenous catheter insertion knowledge, confidence, and skills using a simulation-based blended learning program: A randomized trial. Simulation in Healthcare. 2016;**11**(6):376-384

[56] Glover KR et al. A simulation-based blended curriculum for short peripheral intravenous catheter insertion: An industry-practice collaboration. Journal of Continuing Education in Nursing. 2017;**48**(9):397-406

[57] Ray-Barruel G et al. Infusion phlebitis assessment measures: A systematic review. Journal of Evaluation in Clinical Practice. 2014;**20**(2):191-202

[58] Comparcini D et al. Relationship between peripheral insertion site and catheter-related phlebitis in adult hospitalized patients: A systematic review. Professioni Infermieristiche. 2017;**70**(1):51-60

[59] O'Grady NP et al. Guidelines for the prevention of intravascular catheter-related infections. Clinical Infectious Diseases: An Official Publication of the Infectious Diseases Society of America. 2011;**52**(9):e162-e193

[60] Pérez-Granda MJ et al. Effectiveness of a training program in compliance with recommendations for venous lines care. BMC Infectious Diseases. 2015;**15**(1):296

[61] Easterlow D, Hoddinott P, Harrison S. Implementing and standardising the use of peripheral vascular access devices. Journal of Clinical Nursing. 2010;**19**(5-6):721-727

[62] Ball RD et al. Peripheral intravenous catheter infiltration: Anesthesia providers do not adhere to their own ideas of best practice. Journal of Clinical Anesthesia. 2013; **25**(2):115-120

[63] Chiu P-C et al. Establish a perioperative check forum for peripheral intravenous access to prevent the occurrence of phlebitis. The Kaohsiung Journal of Medical Sciences. 2015;**31**(4):215-221

[64] Simmons LE et al. Preventing preterm birth and neonatal mortality: Exploring the epidemiology, causes, and interventions. Seminars in Perinatology. 2010;**34**(6):408-415

[65] Zenk KE, Dungy CI, Greene GR. Nafcillin extravasation injury: Use of hyaluronidase as an antidote. American Journal of Diseases of Children. 1981;**135**(12):1113-1114

[66] Thigpen J. Peripheral intravenous extravasation: Nursing procedure for initial treatment. Neonatal Network. 2007;**26**(6):379-384

[67] Shenaq SM, Abbase EH, Friedman JD. Soft-tissue reconstruction following extravasation of chemotherapeutic agents. Surgical Oncology Clinics of North America. 1996; **5**(4):825-845

[68] González López JL et al. Indwell times, complications and costs of open vs closed safety peripheral intravenous catheters: A randomized study. Journal of Hospital Infection. 2014;**86**(2):117-126

[69] Kornbau C et al. Central line complications. International Journal of Critical Illness and Injury Science. 2015;**5**(3):170-178

[70] Stevens RJ, Mahadevan V, Moss AL. Injury to the lateral cutaneous nerve of forearm after venous cannulation: A case report and literature review. Clinical Anatomy. 2012;(5):**25**, 659-662

[71] Kim HJ, Park SK, Park SH. Upper limb nerve injuries caused by intramuscular injection or routine venipuncture. Anesthesia and Pain Medicine. 2017;**12**(2):103

[72] Lee SK, Wolfe SW. Peripheral nerve injury and repair. JAAOS-Journal of the American Academy of Orthopaedic Surgeons. 2000;**8**(4):243-252

[73] Kline DG. Surgical repair of peripheral nerve injury. Muscle & Nerve: Official Journal of the American Association of Electrodiagnostic Medicine. 1990;**13**(9):843-852

[74] Campbell WW. Evaluation and management of peripheral nerve injury. Clinical Neurophysiology. 2008;**119**(9):1951-1965

[75] Rickard CM, Ray-Barruel G. Peripheral intravenous catheter assessment: Beyond phlebitis. Lancet Haematology. 2017;**4**(9):e402-e403

[76] Hadaway L. Short peripheral intravenous catheters and infections. Journal of Infusion Nursing: The Official Publication of the Infusion Nurses Society. 2012;**35**(4):230-240

[77] Marsh N et al. Devices and dressings to secure peripheral venous catheters to prevent complications. Cochrane Database of Systematic Reviews. 12 June 2015;(6):cd011070

[78] Rickard CM et al. Securing all intravenous devices effectively in hospitalised patients—The SAVE trial: Study protocol for a multicentre randomised controlled trial. BMJ Open. 2015;**5**(9):e008689-e008689

[79] Jacksson A. Retrospective comparative audit of two peripheral IV securement dressings. British Journal of Nursing. 2012;**21**(suppl 1):S10-S15

[80] Martinez JA et al. Evaluation of add-on devices for the prevention of phlebitis and other complications associated with the use of peripheral catheters in hospitalised adults: A randomised controlled study. The Journal of Hospital Infection. 2009;**73**(2):135-142

[81] Ari Mintz DMSL. Upper extremity deep vein thrombosis-expert analysis. American College of Cardiology. 16 Nov 2017

[82] Duan X et al. Efficacy and safety of nitroglycerin for preventing venous spasm during contrast-guided axillary vein puncture for pacemaker or defibrillator leads implantation. EP Europace. 2013;**15**(4):566-569

[83] Braswell LE. Peripherally inserted central catheter placement in infants and children. Techniques in Vascular and Interventional Radiology. 2011;**14**(4):204-211

[84] Krishnamurthy G, Keller MS. Vascular access in children. Cardiovascular and Interventional Radiology. 2011;**34**(1):14-24

[85] Moyer CD, Gilchrist IC. Transradial bilateral cardiac catheterization and endomyocardial biopsy: A feasibility study. Catheterization and Cardiovascular Interventions. 2005;**64**(2):134-137

[86] Mattox EA. Complications of peripheral venous access devices: Prevention, detection, and recovery strategies. Critical Care Nurse. 2017;**37**(2):e1-e14

[87] Cook LS. Infusion-related air embolism. Journal of Infusion Nursing. 2013;**36**(1):26-36

[88] McCarthy CJ et al. Air embolism: Practical tips for prevention and treatment. Journal of Clinical Medicine. 2016;**5**(11):93

[89] Evans D et al. Complications associated with pulmonary artery catheters: A comprehensive clinical review. Scandinavian Journal of Surgery. 2009;**98**(4):199-208

[90] Jacinto AKdL et al. Flebite associada a cateteres intravenosos periféricos em crianças: Estudo de fatores predisponentes. Escola Anna Nery. 2014;**18**:220-226

[91] Ali J, Summer WG. Chest Radiology: PreTest Self-assessment and Review. United States of America: McGraw Hill Professional; 2001

[92] Cody RJ et al. Sodium and water balance in chronic congestive heart failure. The Journal of Clinical Investigation. 1986;**77**(5):1441-1452

[93] Moffatt-Bruce SD et al. Intravascular retained surgical items: A multicenter study of risk factors. Journal of Surgical Research. 2012;**178**(1):519-523

[94] Wojda TR et al. Foreign intravascular object embolization and migration: Bullets, catheters, wires, stents, filters, and more. In: Embolic Diseases-Unusual Therapies and Challenges. Rijeka: InTech; 2017

[95] Kimberly M, Holt KE. The effectiveness of clinically indicated replacement of peripheral intravenous catheters: An evidence review with implications for clinical practice. Worldviews on Evidence-Based Nursing. 2015;**12**(4):187-198

[96] Webster J et al. Clinically-indicated replacement versus routine replacement of peripheral venous catheters. Cochrane Database of Systematic Reviews. Aug 14 2015;(8): cd007798

[97] Gorski LA, Hadaway L, Hagle M, McGoldrick M, Orr M, Doellman D. 2016 infusion therapy standards of practice. Journal of Infusion Nursing. 2016;**39**(1 Suppl.):S1-S159

[98] Loveday HP et al. epic3: National evidence-based guidelines for preventing healthcare-associated infections in NHS Hospitals in England. Journal of Hospital Infection. 2014;**86**:S1-S70

[99] Gillet J et al. Predictive value of D-dimer assay in superficial thrombophlebitis of the lower limbs. Journal des Maladies Vasculaires. 2007;**32**(2):90-95

[100] Benaya A et al. Relative incidence of phlebitis associated with peripheral intravenous catheters in the lower versus upper extremities. European Journal of Clinical Microbiology & Infectious Diseases. 2015;**34**(5):913-916

[101] Ray-Barruel G et al. Implementing the I-DECIDED clinical decision-making tool for peripheral intravenous catheter assessment and safe removal: Protocol for an interrupted time-series study. BMJ Open. 2018;**8**(6):e021290. DOI: 10.1136/bmjopen-2017-021290

[102] Sen S, Chini EN, Brown MJ. Complications after unintentional intra-arterial injection of drugs: Risks, outcomes, and management strategies. In: Mayo Clinic Proceedings. United States of America: Elsevier; 2005

[103] Lake C, Beecroft CL. Extravasation injuries and accidental intra-arterial injection. Continuing Education in Anaesthesia Critical Care & Pain. 2010;**10**(4):109-113

[104] Shivappagoudar VM, George B. Unintentional arterial cannulation during cephalic vein cannulation. Indian Journal of Anaesthesia. 2013;**57**(3):320-322

[105] Quizlet. Phlebotomy: Tourniquet rationale. 2018. Available from: https://quizlet.com/117376080/phlebotomy-tourniquet-rationale-flash-cards/

[106] Prasarn ML et al. Acute pediatric upper extremity compartment syndrome in the absence of fracture. Journal of Pediatric Orthopaedics. 2009;**29**(3):263-268

[107] Authority PPS. Forgotten but not gone: Tourniquets left on patients. Pennsylvania Patient Safety Authority. 2005;**2**:19-21

[108] Oyster N et al. Characterization of a compartment syndrome–like injury model. Muscle & Nerve. 2015;**51**(5):750-758

[109] Giannoudis PV, Dimitriou R, Kontakis G. Compartment syndromes in the lower limb. In: European Surgical Orthopaedics and Traumatology. Berlin, Heidelberg: Springer; 2014. pp. 221-239

[110] Harvey C. Compartment syndrome: When it is least expected. Orthopaedic Nursing. 2001;**20**(3):15-25

[111] Tolentino JC et al. Introductory chapter: Developing patient safety champions. In: Vignettes in Patient Safety. Vol. 2. Rijeka: Intech; 2018

[112] Stawicki SP, Firstenberg MS. Introductory chapter: The decades long quest continues toward better, safer healthcare systems. In: Vignettes in Patient Safety. Vol. 1. Rijeka: Intech; 2017

[113] Cooke M et al. Not "just" an intravenous line: Consumer perspectives on peripheral intravenous cannulation (PIVC). An international cross-sectional survey of 25 countries. PLoS ONE. 2018;**13**(2):e0193436

[114] Larsen E et al. Experiences of peripheral IV insertion in hospital: A qualitative study. British Journal of Nursing. 2017;**26**(19):S18-S25

Chapter 8

Comprehensive and Live Air Purification as a Key Environmental, Clinical, and Patient Safety Factor: A Prospective Evaluation

Stanislaw P. Stawicki, Chad Brisendine, Lee Levicoff,
Frank Ford, Beverly Snyder, Sherrine Eid and
Kathryn C. Worrilow

Additional information is available at the end of the chapter

http://dx.doi.org/10.5772/intechopen.84530

Abstract

Healthcare organizations strive to provide optimal patient experience by improving care quality and enhancing clinical outcomes, while containing associated costs. In the United States, the Center for Disease Control (CDC) estimates that more than 1.7 million people suffer from an infectious complication annually, representing between 5 and 10% of all hospital admissions and costs ranging between $35B and $88B. Most infectious surface fomites originate from air. Consequently, reducing airborne pathogens should be associated with reduced surface fomites. This study represents the first comprehensive evaluation of infectious and aerosolized pathogens and their speciation, location and concentration within a typical hospital setting. The study provides data regarding the relationship between airborne pathogens and air filtration methodologies in the context of the molecular and microbial epidemiology of illness and infections in the clinical setting. The results demonstrated that using a transformational air purification system provided comprehensive remediation of airborne pathogens and significantly reduced surface-oriented infectious fomites. Overall reduction of airborne and surface bacterial and fungal pathogens responsible for illness and infections will result in a reduction of associated illnesses and HAI rates and improved patient care metrics including stay duration and readmission rates. Improvements in these outcome metrics should correlate to risk mitigation and cost avoidance.

Keywords: airborne pathogens, hospital-acquired infections, HAI, patient care, bacterial pathogens, fungal pathogens, air filtration, air purification, hospital, molecular epidemiology, microbial epidemiology, illness, infection, length of stay, readmission rates, clinical outcomes, HEPA, biological particulates, VOC, volatile organic compounds, ambient air quality, viable particulates, nonviable particulates

1. Introduction

In the United States, the Center for Disease Control and Prevention (CDC) estimated that more than 1.7 million people suffer from an infectious complication within the hospital environment annually, representing between 5 and 10% of all admissions [1]. Approximately 99,000 patients afflicted with hospital-acquired infections (HAIs) die each year [2]. The number of estimated patients with an HAI exceeds that of any required reportable disease in the United States, and the number of deaths attributed to HAIs exceeds many of the top ten leading causes of death reported from the US vital statistics [1]. Moreover, the above estimates likely under-represent the true magnitude of the problem due to erroneous reporting and biases inherent to voluntarily reported data.

Apart from the morbidity and mortality associated with HAIs, the estimated healthcare costs range between $35B and $88B annually [3]. The most recent Pennsylvania Healthcare Cost Containment Counsel (PHC4) Report indicated that hospitals and Medicare spent approximately $3B and $400 M, respectively, toward statewide care of patients affected by HAIs during the reporting year of 2010 [4].

The Centers for Medicare and Medicaid Services (CMS) announced in August 2007 that Medicare would no longer cover additional costs associated with many preventable errors, including those considered "never events" [5]. The list of events that should never occur in the healthcare setting has now been expanded to encompass 29 unique serious reportable events. HAIs represent one of the 29 unique "never events" that are no longer reimbursable and may even result in further economic penalties [6, 7].

It is estimated that full societal costs associated with HAIs arising in US acute care hospitals amount to approximately $96–$147 billion annually [8]. The corresponding per-hospitalization incremental cost ranges between $17,070 and $32,176 [8]. Consequently, it can be reasonably extrapolated that a three-room surgical suite, performing 1,000 annual surgeries with a reported 4% infection rate, would realize a cost avoidance savings of between $171,000 and $322,000 per year specific to the surgical suite with only a 1% decline in HAI rates.

Historically, it has been understood that the patient, the healthcare worker, and various surface areas collectively constitute the primary repositories of pathogens responsible for majority of HAIs [9]. To that end, infection control protocols, in-room sterilization techniques, patient preparation, and hand-washing protocols have been implemented in most hospitals and have been helpful in reducing overall HAI rates [10]. Moreover, recent literature suggests that a significant proportion of pathogens responsible for HAIs are airborne [11]. The Aire~HCX™ (LifeAire Systems, Allentown, Pennsylvania) [12] was specifically designed to comprehensively address these airborne pathogens (AP) as they are inherently generated during routine clinical operations. In environments where Aire~HCX™ is employed, infectious APs are remediated in both the supply and return air before entering the clinical space.

The LifeAire Systems' advanced air purification technology (LAS-APS) exceeds the limitations associated with commonly utilized mechanisms of air filtration [13]. Many in-room sterilization technologies require that the clinical space be vacated before use, leading to temporary loss of functional space. The in-room approaches also provide a "static" clean at the exact time of use [14, 15]. Reentry of patients and healthcare workers and the initiation of clinical processes inherently serve as a source of rapid re-establishment of pathogen populations [16–18]. Unlike the "static" clean model of many of the in-room units, the LAS-APS provides real-time remediation of APs as they are generated during clinical operation. In addition, unlike the "capture" model of the commonly used HEPA filters, the LAS-APS uses a "kill" model and is mathematically and genomically modeled to destroy the DNA and RNA of all bacteria and viruses such that they are rendered noninfectious. HEPA filtration is based upon the capture of viable biological particulates, allowing the spores to grow and proliferate above the space being protected. Air flowing over the spores can disturb and dislodge them such that they enter the clinical space [19]. The "kill" mechanisms incorporated into the LifeAire Systems' technology eliminate these possibilities.

LifeAire Systems' Aire~HCX™ purification unit is installed within the healthcare facility's heating ventilation and air conditioning (HVAC) ductwork. The system is designed to deliver ultrapure, contaminant-free air to any clinical environment. Based on over a decade of research, development, and testing, the Aire~HCX™ system has been tested and proven to deliver air that is 99.99% free of any contaminants, with an associated air purity guarantee [12, 13]. In essence, the LAS-APS was designed to remove all airborne biological pathogens and thus enhance patient safety of the intended healthcare environment by reducing HAI incidence rates, as exemplified by the current collaborative effort between LifeAire and St. Luke's University Health Network (SLUHN). With 69–80% of the pathogens responsible for HAIs being airborne at some point, aggressive remediation of all airborne pathogens will provide for improved patient care and outcomes while reducing the financial burden associated with HAIs.

2. Genesis of LAS-APS air filtration paradigm

With more than a decade of clinical research into the critical role of ambient air quality, the principal investigator (KCW) designed, tested, and patented their transformational air purification technology [12, 13]. This work revealed that one of the key factors impacting successful clinical outcomes was that of the ambient air. Current standards and guidelines as stated are inadequate to provide ambient air optimal for the clinical and patient setting. The clinical environment is impacted by events both external and internal to the space in question. The research highlighted the significant contribution made by patients, healthcare workers, and various clinical processes [20]. External environmental events, even those outside of the immediate proximity of a clinical space, were also found to greatly impact positive outcomes [21–28]. By removing airborne chemical and biological pathogens to below-detection levels, the LAS-APS provides unprecedented control over air quality and significant positive impact on clinical outcomes [25–28].

The LAS-APS provides extremely high levels of filtration as it was designed to kill the anthrax spore (e.g., the most difficult biological pathogen to kill) [29]. The technology used in LAS-APS-patented technology has been tested by the National Homeland Security Research Center and by other third parties. Results indicate that the system renders a broad spectrum of pathogens inert and that it virtually eliminates threatening biological pathogens and volatile organic chemicals from the air—to a level of effectiveness not previously commercially available. Because of its effectiveness toward *Bacillus anthracis*, the LifeAire Systems is able to remediate airborne pathogens such as *Clostridium difficile, Aspergillus, Streptococcus, Pseudomonas,* Staphylococcus (including methicillin-resistant variety), smallpox virus, *Mycobacterium tuberculosis*, influenza virus, etc., each representing a consistent threat to both the hospital environment and rates of HAIs [unpublished data].

3. Materials and methods

The design of the current study includes three zones within two medical surgical floors of a SLUHN Allentown hospital campus. The three geographic zones (**Figures 1–3**) include a control floor with air handling unit (CF-AHU) HEPA-filtration remediation, a zone with mixed AHU-HEPA and LifeAire remediation (MIXED) with recirculated air, and a zone with comprehensive LifeAire Systems Air Remediation (LSAR). Within each of these zones, two occupied and active patient rooms were selected for air quality testing. Each of the two rooms was comprehensively evaluated per zone. The patient rooms were chosen such that the effects of elevators/entrances/exits as well as zone barriers would be minimized. Rooms were further chosen to optimize direct comparisons of resulting data. **Table 1** illustrates the zones and rooms evaluated during the study.

During each testing event, one of the two rooms listed were chosen for the complete suite of particulate, biological, and volatile organic compound (VOC) testing. For this study, the two rooms in each zone were considered equivalent. For each specific testing event, room preference was for patient occupancy, followed by consistency within each room between measurements.

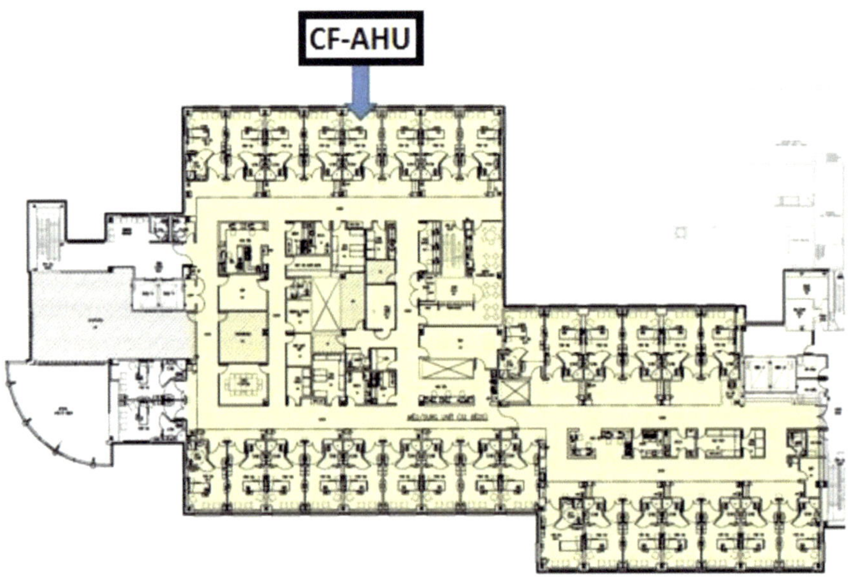

Figure 1. Schematic representing the CF-AHU on the control floor.

Each of the rooms underwent comprehensive evaluation for airborne and surface viable bacterial, fungal, and VOC loads. Three commonly touched patient surfaces and two commonly touched clinical surfaces were evaluated per testing assay (**Tables 2** and **3**). In addition, the final diffuser providing supply air to the patient room and the return vents were swabbed for viable bacteria and fungi (**Table 4**).

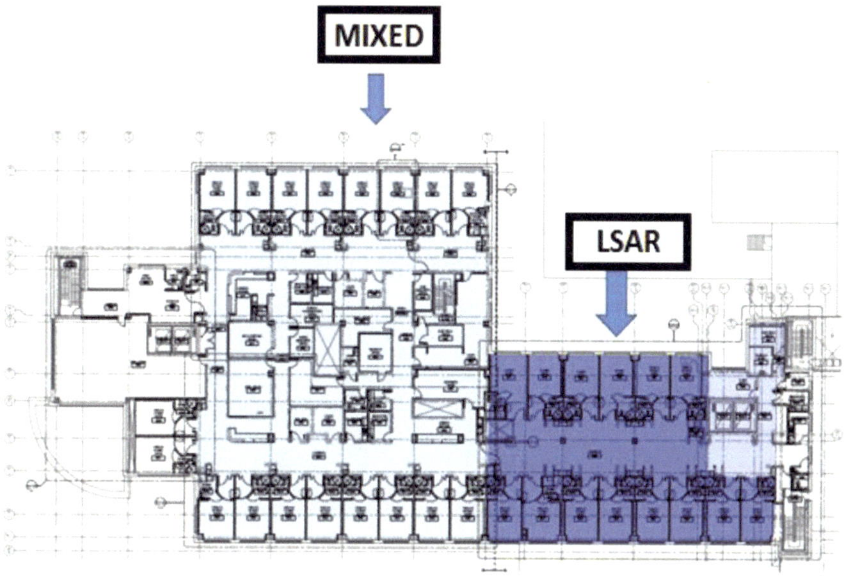

Figure 2. Schematic representing LSAR and MIXED zones, respectively.

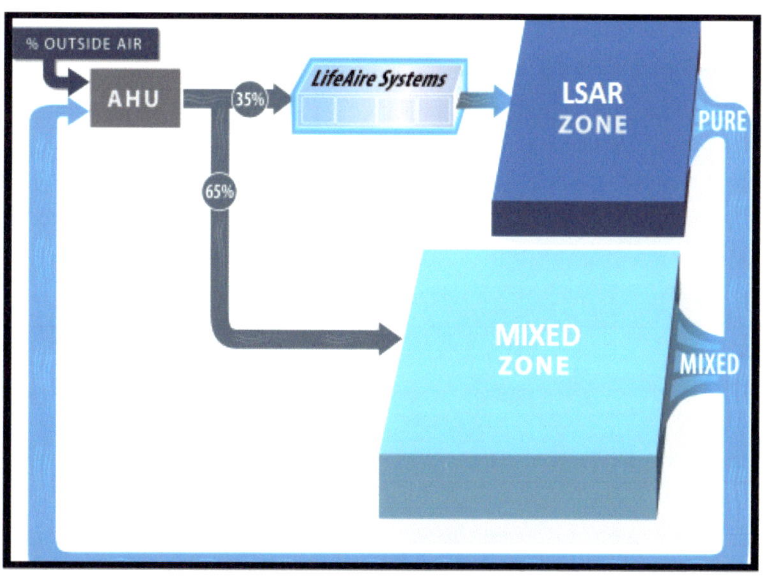

Figure 3. Schematic representation of HVAC layout of the MIXED and LSAR zones.

3.1. Testing assay: viable bacteria by air

Air testing was completed using the third-party laboratories, EMSL, and Galson Laboratories under their proprietary method MICRO-SOP-132 [30, 31]. Following the standard operating procedures (SOPs) provided by the third-party laboratories and using a Viable Andersen Cascade Impactor and calibrated pump, samples were gathered for 5 minutes at 28 liters per minute onto a soy agar plate. The five most concentrated species were then identified and quantified.

3.2. Testing assay: viable bacteria by swab

Surface testing was conducted following all SOPs of the third-party laboratories. Using a sterile swab, an area measuring 2-by-2 inch was sampled in each location with a smooth back-and-forth motion while rolling the swab for 10 seconds. The swab was then capped and sent to the third-party laboratory for testing under method MICRO-SOP-132 [30]. The most prominent five types of bacteria were identified and quantified.

Zone	HVAC design
CF-AHU	AHU-HEPA remediation
MIXED	AHU-HEPA and LifeAire systems remediation
LSAR	LifeAire systems air remediation

Table 1. HVAC design by study zone.

Bedside table (directly in front of patient)
IV support pole/IV support pole
Patient remote control—number buttons

Table 2. Patient surface sampling sites.

IV control faceplate
Pressure cuff bulb

Table 3. Clinical surface sampling sites.

HVAC room diffuser
HVAC room return

Table 4. HVAC surface sampling sites.

3.3. Testing assay: viable fungi by air

Air testing was completed using a third-party laboratory under their proprietary method MICRO-SOP-202 [30]. Following the SOPs provided by the third-party laboratories and using a Viable Andersen Cascade Impactor and calibrated pump, samples were gathered for 5 minutes at 28 liters per minute onto a MEA agar plate. The five most concentrated species were identified and quantified.

3.4. Testing assay: viable fungi by swab

Surface testing was conducted following applicable SOPs of the third-party laboratories. Using a sterile swab, an area measuring 2-by-2 inches was sampled in each location with a smooth back-and-forth motion while rolling the swab for 10 seconds. The swab was then capped and sent to the third-party laboratory for testing under method MICRO-SOP-202 [30]. The five most prominent species of viable fungi were identified and quantified.

3.5. Testing assay: volatile organic compounds (VOC) testing

The measured VOC load of each room was determined using the methodology described in EPA TO-15 [32]. Using an evacuated container, air was captured for 15 minutes. The TO-15 assay determines VOCs in air collected using specially prepared stainless steel canisters and subsequently analyzed by gas chromatography/mass spectrometry (GC/MS). Due to the live hospital setting and available locations to place the testing cylinder, longer sampling times were considered but not employed due to the risk of sample tampering by unmonitored patients, visitors, and clinical staff.

3.6. Testing assay: nonviable particulate testing

Particulate testing was conducted using a modified NIOSH 0500 method [33]. Sampling was conducted for 5 minutes at each testing site. The environmental testing was completed each month with sampling beginning in the morning and progressing through early afternoon. Clinical, housekeeping, operational staff and patients were blinded to both the study and zone locations to minimize any biases associated with behaviors or perceptions. Cleaning SOPs, patient care operations, patient appointment schedules, visitation, patient dining, and all operations of the floor remained unchanged. Sampling occurred during normal visitations, staff consultations, and meals to allow data acquisition and flow to simulate full hospital operations.

4. Results

The overall study results are presented in **Figure 4** and in **Tables 5–7**. All data were provided by independent third-party laboratories after sampling the air and designated surfaces in each patient room associated with the specific study zone, as outlined in the methodology section. A comprehensive environmental assessment of viable bacterial, fungal, and VOC pathogens was conducted each month and repeated a total of 4 times between March and July of 2018.

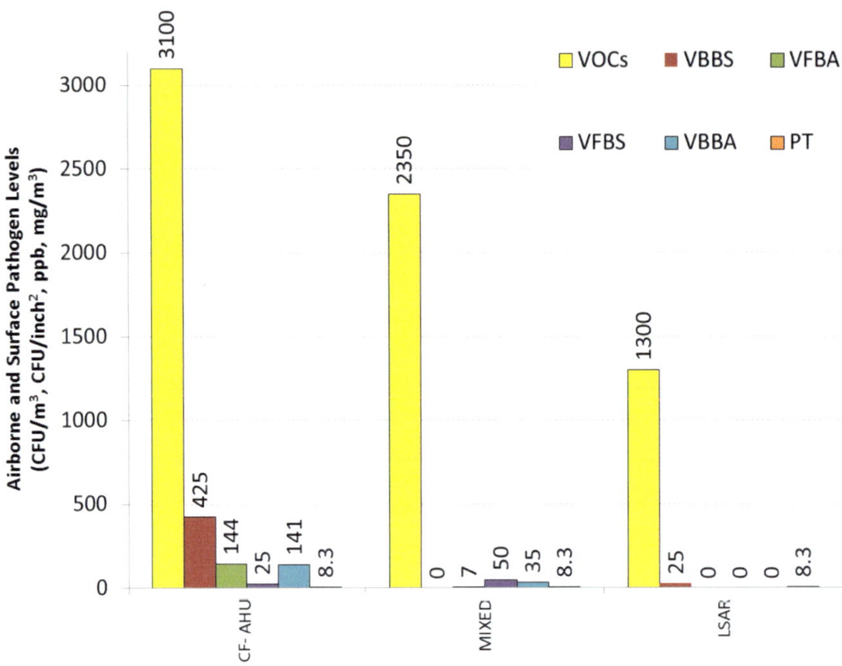

Figure 4. Results for viable airborne and surface bacteria and fungi and VOC load in each zone (CF-AHU, MIXED, and LSAR). Legend: AHU, air handling unit; VFBA, viable fungi by air (CFU/m^3); VFBS, viable fungi by swab (CFU/in^2); VBBA, viable bacteria by air (CFU/m^3); VBBS, viable bacteria by swab (CFU/in^2); VOCs, volatile organic compounds (ppb); PT, particulates (mg/m^3).

Zone	VFBA	VFBS	VBBA	VBBS
CF-AHU	*Aspergillus*	*Aspergillus*	*Micrococcus luteus*	*Micrococcus lylae*
	Cladosporium	*Cladosporium* (remote, return)	*Staphylococcus* spp.: capitis, epidermidis, *haemolyticus, saprophyticus*	Staphylococcus spp.: capitis, *haemolyticus* (remote, return), *hominis, saprophyticus* (return)
			Gram-negative rod	Gram-negative rod (return)
			Bacillus spp.: clausii, licheniformis	Gram-positive cocci (remote, return)
			Dermabacter hominis	
			Kocuria palustris	
MIXED	Yeast	*Rhodotorula* (return)	*Staphylococcus haemolyticus*	Nil
			Bacillus licheniformis	
			Dietzia cinnamea	
			Streptococcus anginosus	

Zone	VFBA	VFBS	VBBA	VBBS
LSAR	Nil	Nil	Nil	*Staphylococcus* spp.: capitis (patient remote), epidermidis (faceplate) *Corynebacterium* (patient remote)

Table 5. Identification of viable bacteria and fungi by air and on surface within the three study zones (CF-AHU, MIXED, and LSAR).

Pathogen	Association with patient illness	Location within clinical space
Aspergillus	Associated with pulmonary infections, infections to skin lesions	Circulating air in patient room Patient remote HVAC Return
Cladosporium	Associated with infections to skin, sinuses, and lungs; significant allergens impacting asthmatics and patients with respiratory diseases; spores produce toxic VOCs	Circulating air in patient room Patient Remote HVAC Return
Staphylococcus saprophyticus	Associated with urinary tract infections	Circulating air in patient room Return
Staphylococcus epidermidis	Skin flora and low association with HAIs	Circulating air in patient room
Staphylococcus capitis	Natural skin flora often associated with infections caused by catheters and aortic valves	Circulating air in patient room Patient Remote HVAC Return
Micrococcus luteus	Source is typically patient-oriented, mouth, mucosae, oropharynx, and upper respiratory tract, often associated with ill patients	Circulating air in patient room
Staphylococcus haemolyticus	Antibiotic resistant and associated with skin flora	Circulating air in patient room Patient Remote HVAC Return
Bacillus clausii	Associated with respiratory infections and GI disorders, produces antimicrobial substances active against *Staphylococcus aureus*, *C. difficile*, and *Enterococcus faecium*	Circulating air in patient room
Bacillus licheniformis	Associated with soil and bird plumage	Circulating air in patient room
Dermabacter hominis	Associated with wound infections, abscesses, and positive blood cultures	Circulating air in patient room

Pathogen	Association with patient illness	Location within clinical space
Kocuria palustris	Pathogen responsible for UTIs	Circulating air in patient room
Gram-positive cocci	*Staphylococcus aureus* and *Streptococcus pyogenes* are two of the most common causes of hospital-acquired pneumonia, septicemia, folliculitis, and surgical site infections	Patient Remote HVAC Return
Gram-negative rods	Associated with *E. coli, Salmonella, Shigella, Pseudomonas*, severe GI illness	Circulating air in patient room HVAC Return
Micrococcus lylae	Associated with skin flora, opportunistic pathogen in immunocompromised patients	HVAC Return
Staphylococcus hominis	Associated with infections in immunocompromised patients	HVAC Return

Table 6. Pathogen characteristics of zone CF-AHU (the control zone).

Pathogen	Association with patient illness	Location within clinical space
Yeast	Associated with pulmonary infections and skin lesion infections	Circulating air in patient room
Rhodotorula	Common clinical contaminant associated with soil and water	HVAC Return
Staphylococcus haemolyticus	Antibiotic resistant and associated with skin flora	Circulating air in patient room
Bacillus licheniformis	Associated with soil and bird plumage	Circulating air in patient room
Dietzia cinnamea	Associated with catheter and orthopedic prosthesis-associated infections in immunocompromised patients	Circulating air in patient room
Streptococcus anginosus	Common cause of abscesses, abdominal and thoracic infections, endocarditis, and bacteremia	Circulating air in patient room

Table 7. Pathogen characteristics of MIXED zone-partial remediation (CF-AHU and 35% LSAR).

Pathogen	Association with patient illness	Location within clinical space
Staphylococcus epidermidis	Skin flora and low association with HAIs	IV control faceplate
Corynebacterium	Normal skin flora, low association with infections, prosthetic devices	Patient Remote
Staphylococcus capitis	Natural skin flora often associated with infections caused by catheters and aortic valves	Patient Remote

Table 8. Pathogen characteristics of LSAR zone patient rooms.

There were 3100 ppb VOCs and <8.3 mg/cubic meter of nonviable particulates in CF-AHU Zone (**Table 6**).

There were no viable bacteria by swab, 2350 ppb VOCs, and <8.3 mg/cubic meter of nonviable particulates in the MIXED Zone (**Table 7**).

Finally, there were no viable bacteria by air, no viable bacteria by swab, no viable fungi by air, 1300 ppb VOCs, and < 8.3 mg/cubic meter of nonviable particulates in LSAR Zone (**Table 8**). The reduction in VOCs is due to the remediation of viable fungal spores and their concomitant production of fungal VOCs. As there was a HEPA filter in place on the serving air handling unit, all air was HEPA-filtered. This was confirmed by the nonviable particulate assessment of <8.3 mg/cubic meter in all study zones.

5. Discussion

Often neglected, indoor air quality is an important component of ensuring healthy and safe environment across various healthcare facilities [34]. It is well established that there exists "strong and sufficient evidence" of the association between ventilation, air movements in buildings, and the transmission of bacterial, fungal, and viral infectious diseases [35]. Consequently, the need for high efficiency/reliable air filtration becomes a necessity, especially in critical environments such as acute care wards, critical care units, isolation units, and operating rooms [36–38]. The current project highlights the importance of an integrated system, such as the LAS-APS, in the modern healthcare environment. The subsequent discussion will synthesize our study's results in the context of acute care hospital setting.

Perhaps most importantly, we noted a substantial decrease in air contaminants across all measurement categories. As the degree of air remediation increased from CF-AHU Zone or the control floor to comprehensive coverage in the patient rooms in LSAR Zone, a significant decrease in airborne bacterial, fungal, and VOC load was observed. The decrease in both bacterial and fungal loads within the air was concomitant with a significant decrease observed on commonly touched clinical and patient surfaces. Within the control zone, many of the pathogens identified in air samples from patient rooms were also found on commonly touched patient surfaces and on the return vents of the room. This data provides a significant contribution to our understanding of the airflow and path of aerosolized pathogens within the typical clinical space.

Previously published data show a strong relationship between the presence of airborne fungal spores and air quality in the hospital setting [39]. As part of the current study, viable fungi species of *Aspergillus* and *Cladosporium* were speciated and quantitated within the control zone patient rooms. Our results demonstrate a substantial decrease in fungal spore detection rates when using LAS-APS technology, as compared to the other approaches.

The presence of bacteria, both in the air and on various surfaces, has been shown to be deleterious to healthcare outcomes [40, 41]. In addition to the fungal species, viable bacterial species were also identified within the patient rooms of the control zone. *Staphylococcus saprophyticus, Staphylococcus epidermidis, Staphylococcus capitis, Micrococcus luteus, Staphylococcus haemolyticus, Bacillus clausii, Bacillus licheniformis, Dermabacter hominis, Kocuria palustris,* Gram-positive cocci, Gram-negative rods, *Micrococcus lylae,* and *Staphylococcus hominis* were found in both the recirculating air of the patient room and on the patient remote and HVAC return. Many of the aerosolized pathogens found within the recirculating air were found on the HVAC return vents. Presence of these pathogens on the return vents confirms their aerosolized nature and threat to the clinical spaces also served by the recirculated air. With the exception of *Bacillus licheniformis,* each of these pathogens is associated with patient illness and infections. The sources of the above airborne pathogens are most likely the patients, visitors, and healthcare workers [42, 43].

It is also important to note that patient rooms in the MIXED Zone received approximately 35% of their recirculated air from the rooms from the LSAR Zone and thus benefited from the installed LAS-APS filtration capacity. The zone also served as an "internal control" as it was located on same the floor as LSAR Zone. Viable yeast was found in the circulating air of the patient rooms in LSAR Zone, and viable *Rhodotorula* was found on the HVAC return vent. Although at a significantly reduced level from that observed in CF-AHU Zone, viable bacteria were identified within the air of the patient rooms of MIXED Zone. *Staphylococcus haemolyticus, Dietzia cinnamea,* and *Streptococcus anginosus,* each a potential source of patient illness and infection, were identified in the patient rooms of MIXED Zone. *Bacillus licheniformis* was also identified but is not associated as a source of patient illness or infection. Interestingly, there were no viable bacteria found on the surfaces swabbed in MIXED Zone. VOCs were reduced over that assessed in CF-AHU Zone. The reduction of viable fungi in MIXED Zone corresponded to the simultaneous reduction in fungal VOC sources.

The patient rooms in LSAR Zone received all of their supply and recirculated air from the LAS-APS installation. There were no viable fungi by air or swab detected in the patient rooms in LSAR Zone. Likewise, there were no viable bacteria by air detected in the patient rooms in LSAR Zone. Low levels of *Staphylococcus epidermidis* were found on the IV control faceplate, and *Corynebacterium* and *Staphylococcus capitis* were found on the patient remote. Because no viable bacteria were identified within the air of the patient rooms in LSAR Zone, the surface bacteria identified on the patient remote and IV control faceplate were most likely due to direct surface-to-surface contact. The lowest levels of VOCs were found in the patient rooms of LSAR Zone as these rooms demonstrated no viable fungi in the circulating air.

The vast majority of infectious surface fomites originate from the air and may be directed onto surfaces by air flow generated by in-room fans and air conditioning systems [44–46]. Consequently, a reduction in airborne bacterial and fungal pathogens should be associated with a reduction in surface fomites [44, 47]. Overall reduction of airborne and surface bacterial and fungal pathogens responsible for patient illness and infections should result in a reduction of associated illnesses, HAI rates, and improved metrics of patient care inclusive of, but not limited to, length of stay and readmission rates. Improvements in these outcome metrics should, by association, correlate to risk mitigation and cost avoidance.

It is important to note that the current, preliminary study represents the first comprehensive evaluation of infectious and aerosolized pathogens and their speciation, location, and concentration within a typical hospital setting. The study provides important data regarding the complex relationship between airborne pathogens and air filtration methodologies in the context of the molecular and microbial epidemiology of illness and infections in the clinical setting. A greater understanding of the role of airborne pathogens in illness in the clinical setting will help facilitate the identification of proper and more optimal levels of remediation.

6. Summary

In the modern healthcare environment, organizations strive to provide optimal patient experience by improving the quality of patient care, enhancing clinical outcomes, while at the same time containing associated costs. Rarely is there an opportunity to utilize technology that positively impacts quality and cost of hospital care without a detrimental "trade off" or major changes in existing behaviors or protocols. We hypothesized that LAS-APS implementation within the SLUHN facility will lead to notable enhancements in air quality across areas serviced by this air filtration/purification system. The current study clearly demonstrates a significant reduction across all forms of air contamination following the installation of LAS-APS. These results represent an important milestone for further research in this critical and often neglected area of healthcare facility operations and maintenance.

Author details

Stanislaw P. Stawicki[1], Chad Brisendine[2], Lee Levicoff[3], Frank Ford[4], Beverly Snyder[5], Sherrine Eid[6] and Kathryn C. Worrilow[7]*

*Address all correspondence to: kcworrilow@lifeaire.com

1 Department of Research and Innovation, St. Luke's University Health Network, Allentown, Pennsylvania, USA

2 Department of Health Information Technology, St. Luke's University Health Network, Allentown, Pennsylvania, USA

3 Department of Planning and Construction Management, St. Luke's University Health Network, Allentown, Pennsylvania, USA

4 Department of Integration, St. Luke's University Health Network, Allentown, Pennsylvania, USA

5 Department of Patient Care Services, St. Luke's University Health Network, Allentown, Pennsylvania, USA

6 Epidemiology and Biostatistics, S.Eid Consulting, Macungie, Pennsylvania, USA

7 LifeAire Systems, Allentown, Pennsylvania, USA

References

[1] Klevens RM et al. Estimating health care-associated infections and deaths in US hospitals, 2002. Public Health Reports. 2007;**122**(2):160-166

[2] Al-Tawfiq JA, Tambyah PA. Healthcare associated infections (HAI) perspectives. Journal of Infection and Public Health. 2014;**7**(4):339-344

[3] Scott RD. The direct medical costs of healthcare-associated infections in US hospitals and the benefits of prevention. 2009

[4] PHC4. 2010 Pennsylvania Healthcare Cost Containment Council Report. 2011. Available from: http://www.phc4.org/dept/dc/ [Accessed: 11-11-2018]

[5] Stawicki SP, Firstenberg MS. Introductory chapter: The decades long quest continues toward better, safer healthcare systems. In: Vignettes in Patient Safety-Volume 1. Rijeka: InTech; 2017

[6] Levinson DR, General I. Adverse Events in Hospitals: National Incidence among Medicare Beneficiaries. Department of Health and Human Services Office of the Inspector General; 2010

[7] Crist J. Never say never: Never events in Medicare. Health Matrix. 2010;**20**:437

[8] Marchetti A, Rossiter R. Economic burden of healthcare-associated infection in US acute care hospitals: Societal perspective. Journal of Medical Economics. 2013;**16**(12):1399-1404

[9] O'Connor C. The impact of healthcare-associated infections on patient care and the role of diagnostic molecular technology in infection prevention and control practice. 2016

[10] Sharpe PA, Schmidt MG. Control and mitigation of healthcare-acquired infections: Designing clinical trials to evaluate new materials and technologies. HERD: Health Environments Research & Design Journal. 2011;**5**(1):94-115

[11] Kowalski WJ. Hospital-acquired infections. HPAC Engineering. 2007

[12] LifeAire_Systems. LifeAire Systems. 2018. Available from: https://lifeaire.com/ [Accessed: 11-11-2018]

[13] LifeAire_Systems. LifeAire Systems: Intellectual Property Summary. 2018. Available from: https://lifeaire.com/intellectual-property/ [Accessed: 11-11-2018]

[14] Pottage T, Walker J. Use of gaseous decontamination technologies for wards and isolation rooms in hospitals and healthcare settings. In: Decontamination in Hospitals and Healthcare. Elsevier; 2014. pp. 299-324

[15] Han JH et al. Cleaning hospital room surfaces to prevent health care–associated infections: A technical brief. Annals of Internal Medicine. 2015;**163**(8):598-607

[16] Weber DJ, Anderson D, Rutala WA. The role of the surface environment in healthcare-associated infections. Current Opinion in Infectious Diseases. 2013;**26**(4):338-344

[17] Dancer SJ. How do we assess hospital cleaning? A proposal for microbiological standards for surface hygiene in hospitals. Journal of Hospital Infection. 2004;**56**(1):10-15

[18] Russotto V et al. Bacterial contamination of inanimate surfaces and equipment in the intensive care unit. Journal of Intensive Care. 2015;**3**(1):54

[19] Price DL et al. Mold colonization during use of preservative-treated and untreated air filters, including HEPA filters from hospitals and commercial locations over an 8-year period (1996-2003). Journal of Industrial Microbiology and Biotechnology. 2005; **32**(7):319-321

[20] Kowalski W. Hospital Airborne Infection Control. Boca Raton: CRC Press; 2012

[21] Worrilow K et al. A retrospective analysis: The examination of a potential relationship between particulate (P) and volatile organic compound (VOC) levels in a class 100 IVF laboratory cleanroom (CR) and specific parameters of embryogenesis and rates of implantation (IR). Fertility and Sterility. 2001;**3**(76):S15-S16

[22] Worrilow KC et al. A retrospective analysis: Seasonal decline in implantation rates (IR) and its correlation with increased levels of volatile organic compounds (VOC). Fertility and Sterility. 2002;**78**:S39

[23] Munch E et al. Poor laboratory air quality and its impact on early embryo development. Fertility and Sterility. 2014;**101**(2):e14

[24] Hall J et al. The origin, effects and control of air pollution in laboratories used for human embryo culture. Human Reproduction. 1998;**13**(suppl_4):146-155

[25] Worrilow K. The Impact of UVC Irradiation on Clinical Pregnancy Rates in an ISO 5 Cleanroom in Vitro Fertilization Laboratory. ASHRAE IAQ; 2009. pp. 4-6

[26] Forman M et al. Statistically significant improvements in clinical outcomes using engineered molecular media and genomically modeled ultraviolet light for comprehensive control of ambient air (AA) quality. Fertility and Sterility. 2014;**102**(3):e91

[27] Esteves SC, Varghese AC, Worrilow KC. Clean Room Technology in ART Clinics: A Practical Guide. CRC Press; 2016

[28] Palter S et al. Multi-center study: Innovative control of ambient air quality in multiple IVF laboratories is associated with statistically significant improvements in clinical outcomes-analysis of 5319 cycles. Fertility and Sterility. 2016;**106**(3):e27-e28

[29] Banerjee D et al. "Green" oxidation catalysis for rapid deactivation of bacterial spores. Angewandte Chemie International Edition. 2006;**45**(24):3974-3977

[30] AIHA. AIHA Laboratory Accreditation Programs, LLC. 2018. Available from: https://www.emsl.com/PDFDocuments/Qualification/AIHA%20EMLAP%20-%20Houston.pdf [Accessed: 12-11-2018]

[31] SGS_Galson. SGS Galson: Industrial Hygiene Lab for Sampling And Analysis. 2018. Available from: https://www.sgsgalson.com/ [Accessed from: 12-11-2018]

[32] EPA. Compendium of Methods for the Determination of Toxic Organic Compounds in Ambient Air, Second Edition: Compendium Method TO-15; Determination Of Volatile Organic Compounds (VOCs) In Air Collected In Specially-Prepared Canisters And Analyzed By Gas Chromatography/Mass Spectrometry (GC/MS). 1999. Available from: https://www.epa.gov/sites/production/files/2015-07/documents/epa-to-15_0.pdf [Accessed: 12-11-2018]

[33] LCS_Laboratory. Total Particulates: Air Sampling by NIOSH 0500. 2018. Available from: http://www.labconserv.com/here/air-testing/industrial-hygiene/particulates-not-otherwise-regulated-niosh-0500-0600-mdhs-144/total-particulates-air-sampling-by-niosh-0500/ [Accessed: 13-11-2018]

[34] Maroni M, Seifert B, Lindvall T. Indoor Air Quality: A Comprehensive Reference Book. Vol. 3. Elsevier; 1995

[35] Li Y et al. Role of ventilation in airborne transmission of infectious agents in the built environment-a multidisciplinary systematic review. Indoor Air. 2007;**17**(1):2-18

[36] Mahieu L et al. A prospective study on factors influencing aspergillus spore load in the air during renovation works in a neonatal intensive care unit. Journal of Hospital Infection. 2000;**45**(3):191-197

[37] O'connell N, Humphreys H. Intensive care unit design and environmental factors in the acquisition of infection. Journal of Hospital Infection. 2000;**45**(4):255-262

[38] MacDonald A. In: White PAF, editor. Protective Air Enclosures in Health Buildings. Pergamon: The Macmillan Press Ltd.; 1981. p. 182. ISBN: 0 333 27678 7£ 15.00

[39] Araujo R, Cabral JP, Rodrigues AG. Air filtration systems and restrictive access conditions improve indoor air quality in clinical units: Penicillium as a general indicator of hospital indoor fungal levels. American Journal of Infection Control. 2008; **36**(2):129-134

[40] Cole EC, Cook CE. Characterization of infectious aerosols in health care facilities: An aid to effective engineering controls and preventive strategies. American Journal of Infection Control. 1998;**26**(4):453-464

[41] Davies A et al. Gaseous and air decontamination technologies for Clostridium difficile in the healthcare environment. Journal of Hospital Infection. 2011;**77**(3):199-203

[42] Beggs C. The airborne transmission of infection in hospital buildings: Fact or fiction? Indoor and Built Environment. 2003;**12**(1-2):9-18

[43] Qudiesat K et al. Assessment of airborne pathogens in healthcare settings. African Journal of Microbiology Research. 2009;**3**(2):66-76

[44] Boone SA, Gerba CP. Significance of fomites in the spread of respiratory and enteric viral disease. Applied and Environmental Microbiology. 2007;**73**(6):1687-1696

[45] Lopez GU et al. Transfer efficiency of bacteria and viruses from porous and nonporous fomites to fingers under different relative humidity. Applied and Environmental Microbiology. 2013;**79**:5728-5734. DOI: 10.1128/AEM.01030-13

[46] Greene V, Bond R, Michaelsen G. Air purification in hospitals. Cleaning and Purification of Air in Buildings. 1960;**797**:16

[47] Eames I et al. Airborne transmission of disease in hospitals. Journal of the Royal Society, Interface. 2009;**6**:S697-S702